# FAM'S MUSCULOSKELETAL EXAMINATION AND JOINT INJECTION TECHNIQUES

# FAM'S MUSCULOSKELETAL EXAMINATION AND JOINT INJECTION TECHNIQUES

**SECOND EDITION**

**GEORGE V. LAWRY, MD, FACP, FACR**
Clinical Professor of Medicine
Chief, Division of Rheumatology
University of California, Irvine
Orange, California

**HANS J. KREDER, MD, MPH, FRCS(C)**
Professor
Departments of Orthopaedic Surgery and Health Policy Management and Evaluation
University of Toronto;
Chief
Holland Musculoskeletal Program;
Marvin Tile Chair and Chief
Division of Orthopaedic Surgery
Sunnybrook Health Sciences Centre
Toronto, Ontario, Canada

**GILLIAN A. HAWKER, MD, MSc**
Professor
Department of Medicine and Health Policy Management and Evaluation
University of Toronto;
Physician-in-Chief of Medicine
Division of Rheumatology
Women's College Hospital
Toronto, Ontario, Canda

**DANA JEROME, MD, MEd, FRCP(C)**
Assistant Professor of Medicine
Division of Rheumatology
University of Toronto
Toronto, Ontario, Canada

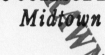
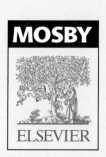

MOSBY

ELSEVIER

MT

# MOSBY
ELSEVIER

1600 John F. Kennedy Blvd.
Ste 1800
Philadelphia, PA 19103-2899

FAM'S MUSCULOSKELETAL EXAMINATION AND
JOINT INJECTION TECHNIQUES

ISBN: 978-0-323-06504-7

**Copyright © 2010 by Mosby, Inc., an affiliate of Elsevier Inc.**

**Library of Congress Cataloging-in-Publication Data**

Fam, Adel G. Musculoskeletal examination and joint injections techniques.
  Fam's musculoskeletal examination and joint injection techniques / [edited by] George V. Lawry ... [et al.]. — 2nd ed.
     p. ; cm.
  Other title: Musculoskeletal examination and joint injections techniques
  Rev. ed. of: Musculoskeletal examination and joint injections techniques / Adel G. Fam, George V. Lawry, Hans J. Kreder. c2006.
  Includes bibliographical references and index.
  ISBN 978-0-323-06504-7
  1. Joints—Diseases—Diagnosis.  2. Joints—Examination.  3. Arthrocentesis. I. Lawry, George V. II. Fam, Adel G. III. Title. IV. Title: Musculoskeletal examination and joint injections techniques.
  [DNLM: 1. Musculoskeletal Diseases—diagnosis.  2. Injections, Intra-Articular—methods.
3. Musculoskeletal Diseases—drug therapy.  4. Physical Examination—methods.  WE 141 F1985 2010]
  RC932.F36 2010
  616.7'2075—dc22                                                                  2010010435

*Acquisitions Editor:* Pamela Hetherington
*Editorial Assistant:* Jessica Pritchard
*Publishing Services Manager:* Hemamalini Rajendrababu
*Project Manager:* Sukanthi Sukumar
*Marketing Manager:* Helena Mutak
*Designer:* Ellen Zanolle

Printed in Canada

Last digit is the print number:  9  8  7  6  5  4  3  2  1

4/1/11

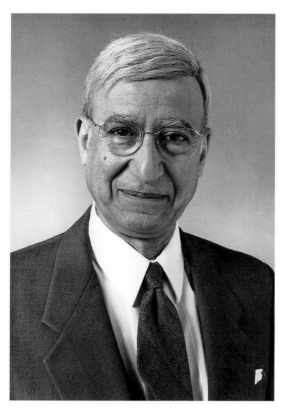

DR. ADEL FAM
October 14th, 1936–April 16th, 2007

Students can often point to a mentor who was a particular
source of inspiration and motivation in their professional
and personal lives.

For those fortunate enough to have been taught by him,
Dr. Adel Fam was that special mentor.

He shared his internationally recognized talents
with skill and passion in an academic career that spanned
over 37 years.

Dr. Fam taught us that a careful history and
physical examination is the most important diagnostic
tool available to clinicians, which can be augmented,
but not supplanted, by blood tests, radiographs, CT scans
and MRI.

This second edition of the project originally begun by
Dr. Fam is dedicated to his memory, and to all those who
share Dr. Fam's enthusiasm for perfecting their clinical
skills to benefit those patients in their care.

# PREFACE

The aim of *Fam's Musculoskeletal Examination and Joint Injection Techniques* is to provide medical students, trainees, rheumatologists, orthopedic surgeons, and other medical practitioners with an accurate, systematic, up-to-date, easily accessible approach to detailed, comprehensive physical examination of the joints and the spine. The text emphasizes pertinent basic anatomy of the joints as it relates to diagnostic accuracy and interpretation of physical signs. Evidence-based critical appraisal of the available literature on physical examination is correlated with the experiences and concepts of the authors, other rheumatologists, orthopedic surgeons, and physiatrists.

The chapters are expertly written, richly illustrated, and both clinically relevant and practical. Each chapter contains a brief description of rheumatic disorders specific to a particular joint. This includes a unique section in the hip and knee chapters on problems following joint replacement arthroplasties. At the end of each section, the techniques of joint and bursal aspiration and injection are discussed with the more common ones demonstrated in accompanying videos.

The diagnosis of rheumatic disorders largely depends on clinical skills and knowledge of applied anatomy. Although musculoskeletal disorders are a common presentation in rheumatologic, orthopedic, and general practices, teaching of joint examination is not sufficiently emphasized in many medical schools and postgraduate residency training programs. Furthermore, in most textbooks of rheumatology, orthopedic surgery, and physiatry, there is limited information about the essential details of basic anatomy, history taking, and principles of joint examination.

A great many people have contributed, directly or indirectly, to the production of this textbook. We are particularly indebted to our colleagues, both junior and senior, teachers, and mentors for their guidance.

Our hope is that this book, written by clinicians for clinicians, will become a useful resource both as a teaching text and a general reference on the basic concepts and techniques of physical examination of the joints and spine. It should benefit not only medical students, trainees, rheumatologists, orthopedic surgeons, and physiatrists but also physiotherapists, occupational therapists, and other health professionals dealing with musculoskeletal disorders.

# CONTRIBUTORS

**CARLO AMMENDOLIA, DC, PhD**
Assistant Professor
Department of Health Policy Management and Evaluation
Faculty of Medicine, University of Toronto;
Chiropractor/ Clinical Researcher
Department of Medicine
Division of Rheumatology, Mount Sinai Hospital
Toronto, Ontario, Canada

**DENNIS BEWYER, PT**
Senior Physical Therapist
University of Iowa
Iowa City, Iowa

**MURRAY J. S. BEUERLEIN, MD, MSc, FRCS(C)**
Orthopaedic Surgeon
Department of Surgery
Red Deer Regional Hospital
Red Deer, Alberta, Canada

**ARTHUR A. M. BOOKMAN, MD, FRCP(C)**
Associate Professor of Medicine
Department of Medicine
Division of Rheumatology
University of Toronto;
Coordinator
Multidisciplinary Sjogren's Clinic
Department of Medicine
Division of Rheumatology
Toronto Western Hospital/ University Health Network
Toronto, Ontario, Canada

**GREGORY W. CHOY, MD, FRCP(C)**
Assistant Professor
Sunnybrook Health Sciences Centre
University of Toronto
Toronto, Ontario, Canada

**ADEL G. FAM†**
Professor Emeritus of Medicine
Sunnybrook and Women's College Health Sciences Centre
Department of Medicine
Division of Rheumatology
University of Toronto
Toronto, Ontario, Canada

**BRUCE V. FREEMAN, DDS, DOrtho, MSc**
Associate in Dentistry
Department of Orthodontics
Faculty of Dentistry
University of Toronto;
Clinician, Headache and Facial Pain Clinic
Department of Dentistry
Mount Sinai Hospital
Toronto, Ontario, Canada

**MICHAEL B. GOLDBERG, MSc, DDS, Dip Periodontology**
Assistant Professor
Faculty of Dentistry
University of Toronto;
Head
Division of Periodontology
Mount Sinai Hospital
Toronto, Ontario, Canada

**ELIZABETH GRIGORIADIS, MD, FRCP(C)**
Lecturer
Department of Medicine
University of Toronto;
Division of Rheumatology
Women's College Hospital
Toronto, Ontario, Canada

**HAMILTON HALL, MD**
Professor
Department of Surgery
University of Toronto;
Orthopaedic Spine Service
Sunnybrook Health Sciences Centre
Toronto, Ontario, Canada

**GILLIAN A. HAWKER, MD, MSc**
Professor
Departments of Medicine and Health Policy Management
  and Evaluation
University of Toronto;
Physician-in-Chief of Medicine
Division of Rheumatology
Women's College Hospital
Toronto, Ontario, Canada

**DANA JEROME, MD, MEd, FRCP(C)**
Assistant Professor of Medicine
Division of Rheumatology
University of Toronto
Toronto, Ontario, Canada

†Deceased

**HANS J. KREDER, MD, MPH, FRCS(C)**
Professor
Departments of Orthopaedic Surgery and Health Policy
 Management and Evaluation
University of Toronto;
Chief
Holland Musculoskeletal Program;
Marvin Tile Chair and Chief
Division of Orthopaedic Surgery
Sunnybrook Health Sciences Centre
Toronto, Ontario, Canada

**GEORGE V. LAWRY, MD, FACP, FACR**
Clinical Professor of Medicine
Chief, Division of Rheumatology
University of California, Irvine
Orange, California

**MICHAEL D. McKEE, MD, FRCS(C)**
Associate Professor of Surgery
University of Toronto;
Adjunct Scientist
Keenan Research Centre
St. Michael's Hospital
Toronto, Ontario, Canada

**HERBERT P. von SCHROEDER, BSc, MD, MSc, FRCS(C)**
Associate Professor
Department of Surgery
University of Toronto;
Medical Director
Hand Program, Rehabilitation Solutions
Toronto Western Hospital
University Health Network
Toronto, Ontario, Canada

**DAVID J. G. STEPHEN, BSc, MD, FRCS(C)**
Orthopaedic Surgeon
Division of Orthopaedic Surgery;
Medical Director
Orthopaedic Trauma
Sunnybrook Health Sciences Centre
Toronto, Ontario, Canada

**HOWARD C. TENENBAUM, DDS, Dip Periodontology, PhD, FRCD(C)**
Professor of Periodontology
Faculty of Dentistry, Laboratory Medicine
 and Pathobiology
Faculty of Medicine
University of Toronto;
Head
Division of Research
Department of Dentistry
Mount Sinai Hospital
Toronto, Ontario, Canada;
Professor of Periodontology
Faculty of Dentistry
Tel Aviv University
Tel Aviv, Israel

# CONTENTS

# ANATOMY OF JOINTS, GENERAL CONSIDERATIONS, AND PRINCIPLES OF JOINT EXAMINATION

George V. Lawry • Dennis Bewyer

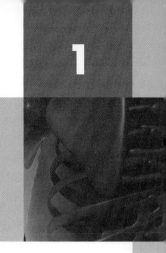

## Applied Anatomy

### TYPES OF JOINTS

Skeletal joints, the sites of articulation between one bone or cartilage and another, are generally of three types: *fibrous joints* (skull-type sutures), *cartilaginous and fibrocartilaginous joints* (discovertebral joints), and *synovial joints* (most limb joints).

**Fibrous joints,** or skull-type articulations, are called **synarthroses:** one bone is joined to another by an unossified fibrous membrane or residual plate of cartilage. Fibrous joints, such as skull sutures, allow little or no movement. Bones united by ligamentous attachments, such as the proximal and distal tibiofibular joints and the superior sacroiliac joints, are called **syndesmoses.**

**Cartilaginous joints** are **amphiarthroses** and are of two types: *fibrocartilaginous* and *cartilaginous.* Bony surfaces coated with hyaline cartilage and united by fibrocartilaginous disks are **symphyses** (fibrocartilaginous joints). Examples include discovertebral, manubriosternal, xiphisternal, and costosternal joints and symphysis pubis. United epiphyseal hyaline cartilage is an example of a cartilaginous amphiarthroidal joint. Amphiarthroses allow a limited range of movement but provide considerable stability.

**Synovial joints** or **diarthroses** are freely movable joints. The bony surfaces are coated with hyaline cartilage and united by a fibrous articular capsule. The synovial membrane lines the inner surface of the capsule but does not cover the articular cartilage (Figure 1-1). The capsule is strengthened by collateral ligaments. Synovial joints comprise most of the joints of the extremities and are the most accessible joints to direct inspection and palpation. Synovial joints share important structural components: subchondral bone, hyaline cartilage, a joint cavity, synovial lining, articular capsule, and supporting ligaments.

**Synovial joints** serve a variety of functions and differ in configuration, permitting specific movements while restricting others. Synovial joints can be subdivided into seven major types:

1. **Spheroidal** (ball-and-socket) joints are universal joints that permit multiaxial movements. Examples include the hip and shoulder.
2. **Ellipsoid** (oval-and-socket) joints are shallower articulations that allow movements in at least two planes. Examples include the wrist, metacarpophalangeal, and metatarsophalangeal joints.
3. **Hinge** joints with interlocking concavity and convexity permit movements in only one plane, such as flexion and extension. The elbow, ankle, and interphalangeal joints of the fingers and toes are hinge joints.
4. **Condylar** joints are characterized by two spheroidal bony condyles articulating with two concave condyles. Examples include the knee and temporomandibular joints.
5. **Gliding or planar** joints are flat or slightly curved joints that only allow sliding or gliding movements. The intercarpal and intertarsal joints are planar joints.
6. **Pivot, trochoid, or axial** (ring-and-pin) joints permit rotation around a central axis. The proximal radioulnar joint and the atlantoaxial joint (C1/C2) are trochoid joints.
7. **Sellar** (saddle-shaped) joints, such as the first carpometacarpal joint, permit flexion, extension, abduction, adduction, and circumduction.

### STRUCTURE OF SYNOVIAL JOINTS AND SUPPORTING TISSUES

The **articular cartilage** is an avascular, aneural, resilient, low-friction, load-bearing tissue covering the articulating bony surfaces. It is capable of absorbing impact by virtue of its compressibility, elasticity, low hydraulic permeability, and self-lubrication (squeeze-film hydrodynamic lubrication). It derives its nourishment through diffusion from the synovial fluid that bathes its surface.

The **synovial membrane** provides an unobtrusive, flexible, low-friction, well-lubricated lining for diarthrodial joints, tendon sheaths, and bursae. Histologically the synovium consists of two layers: an *intimal* or *synovial lining cell layer*—made up of one to three layers of cells or *synoviocytes*—and a *subintimal* or *subsynovial layer* of loose, vascular, fibro-fatty connective tissue. Synovium has important phagocytic functions and produces synovial fluid. Table 1-1 shows different types of synovial effusions.

Joint capsules, ligaments, and tendons are dense fibrous tissues with a major role in musculoskeletal function. Collectively they allow and guide joint motion while resisting high tensile loads without deformation. Laxity or adaptive shortening of these structures affects joint motion and may lead to injury (see Figure 1-1).

**Joint capsules** attach around articular surfaces to form a continuous envelope for the joint. Capsular cells are predominantly fibroblasts with a dense fibrous matrix

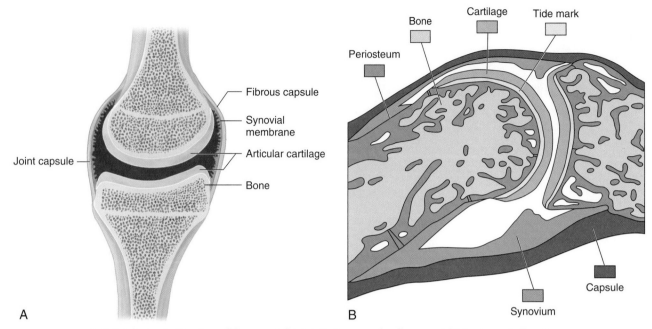

**FIGURE 1-1** **A,** Structure of the synovial joint. **B,** An example of a synovial joint in sagittal section.

| TABLE 1-1 | | | | |
|---|---|---|---|---|
| **TYPES OF SYNOVIAL EFFUSIONS** | | | | |
| | **Noninflammatory** | **Inflammatory** | **Septic** | **Hemorrhagic** |
| Color | Colorless/straw colored | Yellow | Yellow/green | Red |
| Clarity | Transparent | Opaque | Opaque | Opaque |
| Viscosity | High | Reduced | Reduced | Variable |
| WBC count | $< 2000/mm^3$ | $> 2000-100,000/mm^3$ | $> 50,000-100,000/mm^3$ | Variable |
| Differential | $< 25\%$ PMNs | $> 25\%-50\%$ PMNs | $> 90\%$ PMNs | Variable |
| Culture | Negative | Negative | Positive | Variable |

WBC, white blood cell count; PMN, polymorphonuclear leukocytes

surrounding them. The capsule is lined with synovium that provides lubrication for the joint. **Ligaments** attach bone to bone and function to stabilize adjacent bones by restricting abnormal movements. Ligaments may be *intracapsular, capsular,* or *extracapsular,* and they share similar cell and matrix characteristics with the joint capsule and tendon tissues.

The **anterior cruciate ligament (ACL)** is an intracapsular ligament that connects anterior aspect of intercondylar eminence of tibia with medial surface of lateral femoral condyle.

The **medial (tibial) collateral ligament (MCL)** is a capsular ligament connecting the medial epicondyle of the femur with the medial surface of the medial tibial condyle; it is continuous with the capsule and is essentially a thickening of the capsule.

The **lateral (tibial) collateral ligament (LCL)** is an extracapsular ligament, not part of the fibrous capsule of the knee; it connects the lateral epicondyle of the femur with the fibular head.

**Tendons** vary in size and shape, but all attach muscles to bone to transmit the force of muscle contraction to bone. Maintaining tendon tension plays a role in homeostasis of the tendon. Overuse and repetitive trauma results in degenerative changes that outweigh the regenerative process and weaken the tendon.

## General Considerations and History

The patient's history is the essential first step in all musculoskeletal diagnoses, and it focuses on the physical examination. Since diagnosis of nearly all musculoskeletal problems relies upon demonstrating objective findings, the physical examination is enormously important. Despite this, the musculoskeletal examination is often poorly understood and inadequately performed by physicians at all levels of training. Without the ability to perform a proper physical examination, your use of additional diagnostic laboratory testing may be excessive, expensive, and lacking the precision that only comes from recognizing important musculoskeletal physical findings.

### CATEGORIES OF MUSCULOSKELETAL PROBLEMS

Musculoskeletal problems and rheumatic diseases can be practically classified into five major categories, defined by the tissues predominantly affected: *periarticular, articular, bone, nerve,* and *extraarticular.*

**TABLE 1-2**

## MUSCULOSKELETAL PROBLEMS AND RHEUMATIC DISEASES, AFFECTED TISSUES, AND PATTERNS OF INVOLVEMENT

**Periarticular (Soft-Tissue Problems)**

Bursitis, tendinitis
Capsular, ligamentous sprain
Muscular strain

**Articular (Synovial and Cartilaginous Joints)**

Osteoarthritis
Rheumatoid arthritis
Spondyloarthritis
Crystalline arthritis
Infectious arthritis

**Bone**

Trauma
Osteoporosis
Avascular necrosis
Infection
Tumor

**Nerve**

Radiculopathy
Entrapment
Neuroarthropathy
Complex regional pain syndromes
Fibromyalgia (generalized musculoskeletal pain)

**Extraarticular (Systemic Connective Tissue Diseases)**

Systemic lupus erythematosus
Antiphospholipid (anticardiolipin) antibody syndrome
Sjögren syndrome
Polymyalgia rheumatica
Systemic vasculitis
Inflammatory myopathy
Sclerodermatous diseases (skin and fascia)

At each point in your evaluation—as you gather essential historical, physical, and selected laboratory information—ask what tissues are primarily affected. Thinking of musculoskeletal problems in this way provides a useful framework for organizing clinical information. Recognizing the pattern of predominant tissue involvement then directs your attention toward well-defined members of each category, helping to organize your differential diagnosis (Table 1-2).

## CHARACTERISTICS OF MUSCULOSKELETAL PAIN

Pain in nearly any location can be well delineated using the mnemonic **OPQRST**, where O = onset, P = precipitating (and ameliorating) factors, Q = quality, R = radiation, S = severity, and T = timing. This information, combined with the pattern of joint involvement, is helpful in narrowing the preliminary differential diagnosis. The number of joints involved (monoarticular, oligoarticular, or polyarticular); the presence of symmetry or asymmetry; peripheral versus axial joint involvement; small and/or large joint involvement; and a fixed, migratory, or additive pattern of evolution of arthritis are all important features of clinical pattern recognition. Careful questioning about any past joint complaints may supply missing data relating to the location of

prior articular problems and the time course and pattern of evolution of previous musculoskeletal symptoms and signs.

### Onset and Evolution of Symptoms

Knowing the pattern of onset, location, and evolution of articular symptoms is essential for diagnosing musculoskeletal problems. The onset and evolution of articular symptoms in hours to several days is characterized as **acute arthritis** (e.g., crystalline, acute bacterial arthritis). Persistence of symptoms and signs for longer than 6 weeks is characterized as **chronic arthritis** (e.g., osteoarthritis, rheumatoid arthritis), and intermediate duration from days to weeks is referred to as **subacute arthritis.** The pattern of onset and evolution of articular symptoms and signs allows you to direct diagnostic suspicion to certain groups of conditions and eliminate others from serious consideration.

### Patterns of Involvement

A critical feature in clinical diagnosis is the distinction between **arthralgia** (subjective joint pain) and **arthritis** (objective joint swelling or impaired function). Demonstration of objective joint swelling (bony or synovial) on examination is required to make a secure diagnosis of arthritis.

The distribution of joint involvement is one of the most essential aspects of pattern recognition in patients with arthritis. **Monoarthritis** describes involvement of a single joint, **oligoarthritis** (pauciarthritis) involvement of two to four joints, and **polyarthritis** involvement of five or more joints. **Peripheral** and **axial** describe predominant extremity (distal) and spinal (central) joint involvement. **Symmetric** versus **asymmetric** describes whether involvement of joint pairs is bilateral or unilateral. **Small joint** (joints of the hands and feet) and/or **large joint** (shoulder, hip, knee) involvement has considerable diagnostic significance.

Although the presence of pain and tenderness may initially suggest arthritis, **periarticular structures** such as **bursae, ligaments, and tendons** may be responsible for the symptoms and are very important to correctly identify. The term **enthesitis** or **enthesopathy** describes inflammation or abnormality at the insertion site of tendons, ligaments, or joint capsules into bone. This is a particularly prominent clinical feature of spondyloarthropathies, such as ankylosing spondylitis and psoriatic arthritis.

In addition, **muscles** may play a critical role in musculoskeletal symptom development. Throughout day-to-day work and leisure activities, muscles must adapt to sustained positions (sitting, standing, etc.) and repetitive motion that occurs in these adapted postures. As a result, some muscles may become too short and others too long. Some muscles may become hypertrophied from repetitive use, and others become atrophied from disuse. Invariably, substitution for weak muscles by other muscles occurs, and faulty motor patterns develop that lead to compromise of normal joint mechanics. Tendinitis, bursitis, and eventually osteoarthritis may result from this deviation from optimal kinesiology. Restoration of correct muscle length, strength, and motor control is essential to prevent joint injury.

For instance, in the shoulder girdle, supraspinatus function is necessary to produce normal rotation of the humeral head on the glenoid fossa during abduction.

Supraspinatus weakness results in substitution by the deltoid, a large muscle much farther away from the center of rotation of the humeral head. Preferential use of the deltoid muscle in abduction results in superior gliding of the humeral head, producing an impingement syndrome with tendinitis, bursitis, rotator cuff tears, and arthritis.

### Inflammatory Versus Noninflammatory Conditions

Identifying whether articular symptoms suggest an inflammatory or noninflammatory (mechanical or degenerative) process is an important initial step in evaluating musculoskeletal problems. The terms *morning stiffness* and *gelling* are descriptors that help define these distinctions. **Morning stiffness** is the sense of loss of free motion or a slowed, stiff range of movement encountered upon first awakening after sleep. A **gel** or **gel phenomenon** is a similar sense of stiffness following shorter periods of inactivity, such as sitting or resting during the day. **Inflammatory conditions** are usually associated with significant morning stiffness and gelling following inactivity, and this inflammatory pain and stiffness characteristically improves with activity. The duration of morning stiffness may correlate roughly with the severity of inflammation. Morning stiffness of longer than 60 minutes duration is inflammatory in character.

**Noninflammatory (degenerative or mechanical) conditions** are most often accompanied by less than 30 minutes of stiffness and a relatively short gel phenomenon following inactivity. Noninflammatory mechanical pain, such as knee osteoarthritis, usually improves with rest and worsens with activity.

### Extraarticular and Systemic Features

A rapid **rheumatologic review of systems** may reveal important extraarticular or systemic features of musculoskeletal problems not appreciated in the initial history (e.g., fever, photosensitivity, conjunctivitis, Raynaud phenomenon). This review of systems helps "bracket" the presenting problem in order to completely delineate the clinical picture, and it may provide important diagnostic clues of systemic rheumatic disorders such as systemic lupus erythematosus and vasculitis.

## Physical Examination

### ESSENTIAL CONCEPTS

A central axial spine, paired peripheral joints, and symmetric musculature provide the basis for essential **side-to-side comparison** during the musculoskeletal examination. Recognizing **asymmetry** is important and may provide an initial clue in diagnosing an abnormality.

Both active and passive ranges of motion are important in assessing joint function. **Active range of motion** is patient-initiated movement of the joint that tests integrated function and requires intact innervation, muscle and tendon function, and joint mobility. **Passive range of motion** is examiner-initiated movement of a joint and tests only joint mobility. The combined use of passive as well as active range of motion minimizes the need for patient instruction and maximizes the speed and efficiency of the exam (Figure 1-2). Whenever joint movement is anticipated to be painful, it is best to first observe active range of motion (patient-initiated movement) to appreciate the degree of pain and dysfunction before gently attempting passive range of motion (examiner-initiated manipulation).

### Importance of Objective Findings

**Joint tenderness** is at least in part a subjective reaction (joint tenderness ≠ arthritis). The location of tenderness may be helpful in distinguishing an articular problem (joint-line tenderness) from periarticular problems (bursitis, tendinitis) where more localized tenderness is found over a lesion. Tenderness must be correlated with the finding of an objective, visible, or palpable abnormality for a diagnosis of arthritis to be made.

**Joint redness,** or **erythema,** is an objective abnormality and depends on the acuteness and severity of the underlying inflammation. When present, significant erythema may suggest the possibility of infection or crystalline arthritis.

**Joint warmth** is also an objective finding and depends on the acuteness and severity of the underlying inflammation. When present, joint warmth can be a very helpful clinical sign of arthritis. (Clinically important chronic inflammation, however, is often cool to palpation, as frequently seen in chronic rheumatoid arthritis.)

**Joint swelling** is an extremely important and definitive clinical sign. Swelling due to synovial fluid (joint effusion) or

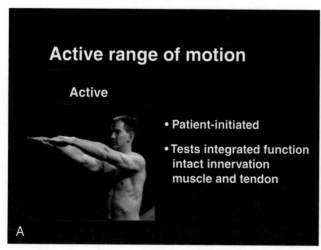

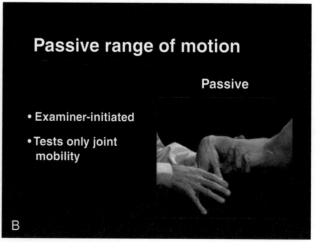

**FIGURE 1-2  ACTIVE AND PASSIVE RANGE OF MOTION.**

swollen synovial tissue (synovial membrane inflammation = synovitis) provides the clinician with definitive evidence of the presence of arthritis. Swelling due to bony enlargement (osteophytes) is also an extremely important physical finding, indicating the presence of underlying primary or secondary osteoarthritis.

**Crepitus** refers to a "grating" sensation felt under the examiner's hand during joint movements, and it may indicate roughening of the cartilaginous surface (*cartilaginous crepitus*) or complete loss of hyaline cartilage with bone-on-bone contact (*bony crepitus*).

**Joint damage and deformity** are important, usually permanent, signs of prior injury (ligamentous laxity, tendon rupture, flexion contracture) or arthritis (ulnar deviation, subluxation). The pattern of such damage and deformity can provide important clinical clues to the underlying process.

**Manual muscle testing** is an important part of the physical examination of musculoskeletal conditions. Careful evaluation of muscle length and strength provides valuable information regarding diagnosis, the focus of rehabilitation, and a basis for determining progress. The art and science of manual muscle testing involves specific positioning to isolate a muscle, test it in its shortest position, and grade its strength on a scale from 0 to 5. For instance, grade 3 strength means the patient can hold the test position against gravity but not with any other pressure applied. Manual muscle testing is the tool of choice for evaluating muscle imbalances.

## EXAMINATION COMPONENTS

There are four essential steps in the examination of joints: *inspection, palpation, active and passive range of motion,* and *the assessment of supporting structures and special testing.* Inspect the joint for asymmetry, erythema, swelling, and deformity. Palpate for tenderness; warmth; synovial thickening; effusion (in inflammatory synovitis); bony, osteophytic swelling (in primary and secondary osteoarthritis); and crepitus. Take the joint through a combination of active (patient-initiated) and passive (examiner-initiated) range-of-motion tests appropriate to the specific joint. Finally, assess supporting structures—such as ligaments, tendons, and muscles—and perform special testing using regional evaluations specific to particular joints. Examples of special testing include manual muscle testing, impingement testing (shoulder), and testing for Tinel sign (entrapment neuropathies).

### Recording Exam Findings

A brief record of abnormalities can be made by organizing your examination into the following categories: **upper extremities** (fingers, wrists, elbows, and shoulders); **lower extremities** (hips, knees, ankles, and feet); **spine** (cervical, thoracic, lumbosacral, and sacroiliac joints); and **gait** (noting uneven rhythm, limp, and asymmetry). Abnormalities such as tenderness, swelling, altered range of motion, and deformity can then be easily reviewed and compared by subsequent examiners.

For example, a patient with *significant generalized, primary osteoarthritis* might have a joint examination record as follows:

**Diagram for Recording Joint Disease Activity**

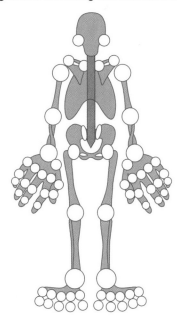

**FIGURE 1-3    DIAGRAM FOR RECORDING MUSCULOSKELETAL EXAM FINDINGS.**

**UE:** multiple Heberden nodes; mild tenderness and cool swelling; R second and fourth and L fifth PIPs; subluxation and "squaring" of first CMCs; nontender acromioclavicular osteophytes.

**LE:** R hip: flexion 90°, ER 40°, IR 10° with groin pain at end IR; L hip: flexion 120°, ER 60°, IR 40° and painless; bilateral hallux valgus.

**C SPINE:** mild ↓ flexion; 40° R and L rotation; ↓↓ extension with mild pain posteriorly.

**LS SPINE:** full flexion; ↓ lateral bend; ↓↓ extension with pain at lumbosacral junction without radiation.

**GAIT:** antalgic gait with R groin discomfort.

Use of cartoon diagrams to record findings can also be quite helpful (Figure 1-3).

## SELECTED READINGS

Agur, A.A., Dalley, A.F., 2004. Grant's Atlas of Anatomy, eleventh ed. Lippincott Williams & Wilkins, Philadelphia.

Grant, J.C.B., 1989. Grant's Method of Anatomy: A Clinical Problem-Solving Approach, eleventh ed. Lippincott Williams & Wilkins, Philadelphia.

Griffin, L.Y. (Ed.), 2005. Essentials of Musculoskeletal Care, third ed. American Academy of Orthopedic Surgeons, Rosemont, IL.

Hoppenfeld, S., 1976. Physical Examination of the Spine and Extremities. Appleton-Century-Crofts, New York.

Kendall, F.P., 2005. Muscle Testing and Function, fifth ed. Lippincott Williams & Wilkins, Philadelphia.

Klippel, J.H. (Ed.), 2008. Primer on the Rheumatic Diseases, thirteenth ed. Springer-Arthritis Foundation, Atlanta, GA.

Sahrmann, S.A., 2002. Movement Impairment Syndromes. Mosby, St. Louis.

Weinstein, S.L., Buckwalter, J.A., 2005. Turek's Orthopedics, sixth ed. JB Lippincott, Philadelphia.

# 2

# THE SHOULDER

Murray J. S. Beuerlein • Michael D. McKee • Adel G. Fam

## Applied Anatomy

Shoulder movements are a synthesis of motion at four artic-ulations: *sternoclavicular, acromioclavicular, glenohumeral,* and *scapulothoracic.*

### STERNOCLAVICULAR JOINT

The **sternoclavicular** (SC) **joint** is a spheroidal joint between the medial end of the clavicle and both the manubrium and the first costal cartilage. An intraarticular fibrocartilaginous disk stabilizes the joint and prevents medial displacement of the clavicle. The joint capsule is reinforced by the anterior and posterior SC ligaments.

### ACROMIOCLAVICULAR JOINT

The **acromioclavicular** (AC) **joint** is a spheroidal joint between the lateral end of the clavicle and the acromion pro-cess of the scapula (Figure 2-1). A small, intraarticular fibro cartilaginous disk divides the joint into two compartments. A subcutaneous, noncommunicating bursa may be present over the joint. The stability of the AC joint depends on the capsule and the superior and inferior AC ligaments. The cor-acoclavicular ligament (conoid and trapezoid parts) extends between the distal clavicle and the coracoid process of the scapula (Figure 2-2). It suspends the scapula, stabilizes both the clavicle and the scapula, and maintains a close relation between the two bones during shoulder movements, thus limiting scapular rotation around the AC joint. The AC and SC joints augment the range of shoulder movements, par-ticularly abduction and rotation. The joints also allow slight axial rotation of the clavicle, as well as elevation/depression and forward/backward thrusting of the shoulder.

### GLENOHUMERAL JOINT

The **glenohumeral** (GH) **joint**, the main articulation of the shoulder complex, is a multiaxial, ball-and-socket synovial articulation between the glenoid fossa of the scapula and the humeral head (Figure 2-1). The lax articular capsule and the small area of contact between the shallow glenoid fossa and the spheroidal humeral head permit a wide range of motion. The stability of the joint depends on a number of static and dynamic stabilizers. Static stabilizers include nega-tive intraarticular pressure; GH bone geometry; the capsule; the glenoid labrum; the superior, middle, and inferior GH

ligaments; and the coracohumeral ligament. The capsule, which fuses in part with the tendons of the rotator cuff, has two apertures: one for the long biceps tendon (origin from the supraglenoid tubercle) and one for the subscapularis bursa. The labrum, a ring of fibrocartilage that surrounds and deepens the glenoid cavity, contributes significantly to GH joint stability. Through a bumper effect, it functions as a "chock block" to prevent translational forces.

The inferior GH ligament complex is the primary liga-mentous stabilizer of the abducted GH joint and serves to prevent anteroinferior shoulder dislocation. The middle GH ligament is tensioned at 45° of abduction, and the superior GH ligament is tight in adduction.

Dynamic stabilizers play an important role in the stability of the shoulder. They include two musculotendinous layers: 1) an inner stratum, made of the rotator cuff muscles (supra-spinatus, infraspinatus, teres minor, and subscapularis) and the long biceps tendon (origin from supraglenoid tubercle from glenoid fossa), and 2) an outer stratum, composed of the deltoid, teres major, pectoralis major, latissimus dorsi, and trapezius muscles.

The muscles of the inner stratum stabilize and retain the humeral head in the glenoid cavity during shoulder move-ments (cavity-compression mechanism), while simultane-ously providing abduction (supraspinatus—origin from the supraspinatus fossa of scapula and insertion into the superior part of the greater tuberosity), external rotation (infraspina-tus and teres minor—origin from the infraspinatus fossa and axillary border of the scapula, respectively, and inser-tion into the posterior aspect of the greater tuberosity), and internal rotation (subscapularis—origin from the subscapu-laris fossa and insertion into the lesser tuberosity). At the ini-tiation of shoulder abduction, both the rotator cuff and the long biceps tendon depress and stabilize the humeral head against the glenoid cavity to counteract the upward pull of the more powerful deltoid muscle. The mechanism whereby these two groups of muscles combine to produce abduc-tion, the one (deltoid muscle) elevating and the other (rota-tor cuff and biceps tendons) stabilizing the humeral head, is termed *force-coupling.* The muscles of the outer stratum are the prime movers of the shoulder. These provide abduction, flexion, extension, adduction, and some degree of rotation.

The coracoacromial arch—made up of the coracoid pro-cess, coracoacromial ligament, and acromion—acts as a pro-tective, secondary socket for the humeral head, under which the rotator cuff tendons and long biceps tendon glide, with the subacromial bursa lying in between. The arch prevents

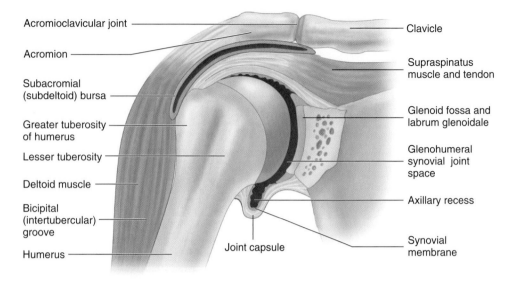

Acromioclavicular joint

Acromion

Subacromial (subdeltoid) bursa

Greater tuberosity of humerus

Lesser tuberosity

Deltoid muscle

Bicipital (intertubercular) groove

Humerus

Joint capsule

Clavicle

Supraspinatus muscle and tendon

Glenoid fossa and labrum glenoidale

Glenohumeral synovial joint space

Axillary recess

Synovial membrane

**FIGURE 2-1   THE SHOULDER.**

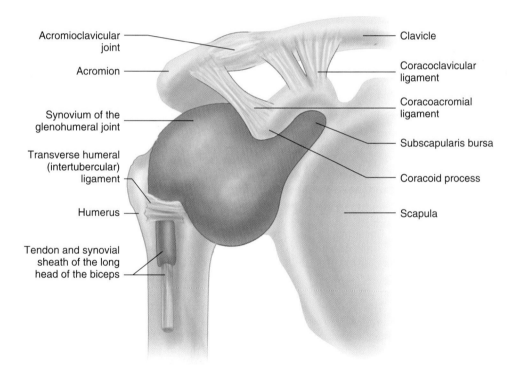

Acromioclavicular joint

Acromion

Synovium of the glenohumeral joint

Transverse humeral (intertubercular) ligament

Humerus

Tendon and synovial sheath of the long head of the biceps

Clavicle

Coracoclavicular ligament

Coracoacromial ligament

Subscapularis bursa

Coracoid process

Scapula

**FIGURE 2-2   THE SHOULDER (SYNOVIAL MEMBRANE AND OUTPOUCHINGS).**

upward displacement of the humeral head and protects the head and rotator cuff from direct trauma. The undersurface of the acromion is commonly flat (type 1); less frequently, it is downwardly curved (type 2) or hooked (type 3), but these conditions are more commonly associated with subacromial impingement.

The synovium of the shoulder lines the inner surface of the capsule. It has two extracapsular outpouchings, the tenosynovial sheath of the long biceps tendon and the bursa beneath the subscapularis tendon (Figure 2-2). A communicating infraspinatus bursa is sometimes present. The subcoracoid bursa lies between the shoulder capsule and the coracoid process, but it rarely communicates with the joint.

## SCAPULOTHORACIC MOVEMENTS

The so-called scapulothoracic articulation is not a true joint but functions as an integral part of the shoulder complex. The scapula, which is connected to the posterior aspect of the chest wall by the axioappendicular muscles, provides the origin for the rotator cuff muscles and deltoid, and the trapezius inserts into its superior aspect. Scapulothoracic movements that include rotation, elevation, depression, protrusion, retraction, and circumduction are important for the normal functioning of the shoulder. The scapulothoracic bursa is located between the serratus anterior and the chest wall, just medial to the inferior angle of the scapula.

## NERVE SUPPLY TO THE SHOULDER JOINT

The shoulder joint derives its nerve supply from three branches of the brachial plexus: suprascapular, axillary, and lateral pectoral nerves (C5/C6). The axillary nerve and the posterior circumflex humeral artery pass through the quadrilateral or quadrangular space, which lies infero-posterior to the GH joint, bounded by the teres minor superiorly, the teres major inferiorly, the long head of triceps medially, and the shaft of the humerus laterally (Figure 2-3).

## SHOULDER PAIN AND HISTORY TAKING

Shoulder pain is a common symptom of diverse causes (Table 2-1). The pain may originate in the GH or AC joint or in periarticular structures, or it may be referred from the cervical spine, brachial plexus, thoracic outlet, or infradiaphragmatic structures. Important points in the history include age, hand dominance, occupational and sport activities involving heavy lifting or overhead repetitive movements, history of trauma, onset, location, character, duration, radiation of the shoulder pain, aggravating and relieving factors, presence of night pain, and the effect on shoulder function. Associated symptoms—shoulder stiffness, restriction of movement, grinding, clicking, instability, or weakness—may also provide useful diagnostic clues.

It is also important to determine whether the shoulder pain is isolated or associated with other stiff, painful, or swollen joints. Shoulder pain may be a feature of a more systemic arthritis. Other joint history, and a history of systemic features, may need to be taken into consideration.

# Common Disorders of the Shoulder

## ROTATOR CUFF PATHOLOGY

The spectrum of rotator cuff pathology ranges from mild rotator cuff tendinopathy to partial and complete rotator cuff tears. If the tear increases in size, a massive rotator cuff tear (< 5 cm) may develop. This can lead to the proximal migration of the humeral head and secondary GH osteoarthritis (cuff tear arthropathy).

Causative factors include repetitive low-grade trauma or unaccustomed activities, excessive overhead use in sport or work, lack of conditioning, aging, and compromise of the rotator cuff space by osteophytes on the undersurface of the AC joint, type 2 or 3 acromion, or an os acromiale (unfused acromial epiphysis). Abnormal tensile stresses that exceed the elastic limits of tendons can lead to cumulative micro-failure of the molecular links between tendon fibrils, called *fibrillar creep*. With aging, tendons become less flexible and less elastic, making them more susceptible to injury and tears. A short-ended musculotendinous unit, from lack of regular stretching exercises, is also prone to injury.

In young persons, rotator cuff tendinopathy is often caused by a sport-related injury; for example, from use of the arm in an overhead position in baseball, racquetball, tennis, or swimming. In older individuals, an antecedent history of repetitive movements above the shoulder level or of strenuous or unaccustomed arm activity is common. Symptoms include aching pain in the shoulder, lateral aspect of the upper arm, and deltoid insertion; pain with movement, particularly abduction and internal rotation; night pain when rolling onto the affected side; restriction of shoulder movements; and sometimes weakness caused by a rotator

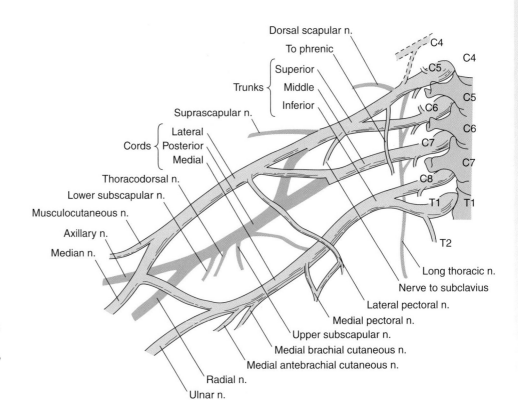

**FIGURE 2-3    ARRANGEMENT OF THE BRACHIAL PLEXUS AND ITS TRUNKS, CORDS, AND TERMINAL BRANCHES.** (From Rockwood CA, Matsen FA, Wirth MA, et al., eds.: *The Shoulder*, 4th ed. Philadelphia: Saunders, 2009.)

TABLE 2-1

## DIFFERENTIAL DIAGNOSIS OF SHOULDER PAIN

**Articular Causes**

GH and AC arthritis: OA, RA, PsA, trauma, infection, crystal-induced
Ligamentous and labral lesions
GH and AC joint instability
Osseous: fracture, osteonecrosis, neoplasm, infection

**Periarticular Causes**

Chronic impingement and rotator cuff tendinitis
Bicipital tendinitis
Rotator cuff and long biceps tendon tears
Subacromial bursitis
Adhesive capsulitis

**Neurological Lesions About the Shoulder**

Thoracic outlet syndrome
Acute brachial plexus neuritis
Quadrilateral space syndrome
Suprascapular nerve entrapment syndrome
Cervical radiculopathy

**Referred and Miscellaneous Causes**

Angina pectoris
Diaphragmatic and infradiaphragmatic disorders: pericarditis, pleurisy, gallbladder disease, subphrenic abscess
Axillary artery or vein thrombosis
Reflex sympathetic dystrophy syndrome and shoulder–hand syndrome
Polymyalgia rheumatica, myositis
Diffuse fibromyalgia and myofascial pain syndrome
Somatization disorder and psychogenic regional pain syndrome

AC, acromioclavicular; GH, glenohumeral; OA, osteoarthritis; PsA, psoriatic arthritis; RA, rheumatoid arthritis

cuff tear. The patient typically experiences shoulder pain on active abduction, especially between 60° and 120°, and difficulty with overhead work, lifting, or reaching behind the back when dressing. Clinical findings include a painful arc between 60° to 120° of abduction, limitation of active movement by pain, and tenderness localized to the rotator cuff and greater tuberosity. The supraspinatus test, Neer impingement test, Neer impingement sign, and Hawkins impingement sign (see Special Tests of Shoulder, p. 13) are often positive.

Rotator cuff tears can be partial or complete, acute or chronic, small or massive. In young adults, acute tears often result from direct trauma or a sport-related injury. In older patients, minor trauma, superimposed on cuff tendon that is already frayed from chronic impingement and age-related attritional changes, can lead to tears.

Clinical features include shoulder pain on abduction, night pain, varying degrees of weakness of abduction and external rotation, local tenderness, wasting of the supraspinatus and/or infraspinatus muscles, and loss of range of motion with difficulty elevating the arm to greater than 90° without shrugging the shoulder (positive shrug sign). The supraspinatus test, Neer impingement sign, and Hawkins impingement sign are usually positive. Rupture of the long biceps tendon may also be present. In complete tears, the drop-arm sign is positive. The diagnosis of rotator cuff tears

can be confirmed by ultrasonography, magnetic resonance imaging (MRI), or arthroscopy.

## BICIPITAL TENDINITIS

Bicipital tendinitis often results from chronic subacromial impingement occurring in association with rotator cuff tendinitis and rotator cuff tears. Primary isolated bicipital tendinitis is rare and develops as an overuse injury resulting from repetitive stresses applied to the tendon in certain sports, such as weight lifting and ball throwing. Anterior shoulder pain that is increased by overhead activities, shoulder extension, and elbow flexion is the main symptom. There is localized tenderness over the tendon in the bicipital groove, the Yergeson sign (see Tests for Biceps Tendon, p. 16) is present, and the speed test is often positive. Passive extension of the shoulder or resisted flexion of the elbow may also reproduce the pain. Signs of chronic impingement and GH instability are often present. Rupture of the long biceps tendon is associated with a positive Popeye sign.

Subluxation of the bicipital tendon is caused by traumatic rupture of the intertubercular (transverse humeral) ligament. It is associated with anterior shoulder pain, a clicking sensation of the shoulder as it "goes out and pops back in," tenderness in the bicipital groove, and a positive transverse humeral ligament test.

## ADHESIVE CAPSULITIS

Adhesive capsulitis, also known as *frozen shoulder,* is characterized by progressive global restriction of shoulder movements and is associated with pain and functional disability. A period of immobility of the shoulder is the most common predisposing factor. The capsulitis may be secondary to shoulder trauma, rotator cuff tendinitis or tears, bicipital tendinitis, or GH arthritis, or it may coexist with diabetes mellitus, hypothyroidism, or cerebrovascular events. An initial synovitis phase is followed by fibrous thickening and contracture of the capsular folds, axillary recess, rotator cuff interval, and coracohumeral ligament. The shortening of the coracohumeral ligament and rotator cuff interval acts as a tight checkrein, limiting external rotation. Capsular adhesions are rare.

The clinical course can be divided into four overlapping stages. In stage I, there is painful limitation of active and passive shoulder movements with diffuse synovitis on both arthroscopy and biopsy. Stage II is a painful "freezing" phase; shoulder pain, tenderness, and progressive, painful, global restriction of movements are present, as well as characteristic limitation of external rotation in the absence of GH arthritis. Synovial inflammation and a tight, thickened capsule are observed on both arthroscopy and biopsy. In stage III, an adhesive or "frozen" phase, there is minimal pain; movements are markedly restricted, and the patient is unable to elevate the arm to 90° without shrugging the shoulder (positive shrug sign). Disuse atrophy of the deltoid and scapular muscles is common. A thickened, contracted capsule and fibrotic synovitis are observed on both arthroscopy and biopsy. In stage IV, a resolution or "thawing" phase, pain is minimal with an increasing range of motion.

Criteria for diagnosis of adhesive capsulitis include an insidious onset, true shoulder pain lasting longer than

3 months, night pain, painful restriction of all active and passive movements with external rotation reduced to less than 50% of normal, and a normal radiologic appearance. Although 90% of patients recover some use of the extremity within 12 to 18 months, about 40% develop more prolonged pain, restriction of movement, and functional disability.

## GLENOHUMERAL INSTABILITY

### Acute Instability

Acute shoulder instability usually results from a traumatic event such as a fall, sports injury, or motor vehicle collision. More than 90% of all acute shoulder instability is anterior. Typically the patient will present with a "squared-off " shoulder on inspection and significant pain with any shoulder motion. A detailed neurovascular exam of the affected limb is essential. Following confirmatory x-rays, a closed reduction of the shoulder is performed.

Acute posterior dislocations are rare but should be considered when there is a history of seizure or electrocution. The arm is usually held in internal rotation, and loss of external rotation is a typical physical exam finding. Closed reduction of this injury is usually successful if the diagnosis is made promptly.

### Recurrent Instability

Most cases of recurrent shoulder instability develop following an initial traumatic shoulder dislocation. A Bankart lesion, a traumatic avulsion of the anterior inferior glenoid labrum, is the essential lesion in this disorder. Patients with recurrent anterior shoulder instability complain of "not trusting" their shoulder when their arm is away from the body. On exam they have a positive anterior apprehension sign and a positive relocation sign. These patents do well with surgical stabilization of the shoulder.

Multidirectional shoulder instability tends to be atraumatic and often bilateral. The history will usually lack a single traumatic episode. Physical exam often shows generalized ligamentous laxity. A sulcus sign is commonly seen. Surgery is not as successful in these patients, and rehabilitation is the mainstay of treatment in recurrent multidirectional shoulder instability.

## TRAUMATIC LESIONS OF THE ACROMIOCLAVICULAR JOINT

Trauma to the AC joint can lead to disruption of the capsule, ligaments, and fibrocartilaginous disk. Local pain, tenderness, swelling, and a painful arc from 90° of abduction upward are the main findings. Pain at the AC joint can be reproduced by passive adduction of the extended shoulder behind the back (adduction stress test) and by abducting the shoulder 90° and then adducting it across the chest at shoulder height, compressing the AC joint (cross-arm AC-loading adduction test).

## ARTHRITIS OF THE SHOULDER

Both inflammatory arthritis, such as rheumatoid arthritis, and degenerative arthritis, such as osteoarthritis, can affect the shoulder joints. Inflammatory arthritis may involve the AC, GH, or SC joint, and the patient may experience swelling and tenderness of the affected joints. The shoulder is painful with range of motion in all directions, and range may be limited. Other synovial joints in the body are often affected, and treatment is generally directed toward the systemic condition.

Primary osteoarthritis is common in the AC joint and less common in the GH joint. In some cases it may occur at the GH joint secondary to an inflammatory process. In osteoarthritis the shoulder is generally painful with activity and may get progressively worse over time. It is painful throughout the range of motion, which is often limited. Crepitus is classically felt over the affected joint.

## NEUROLOGIC LESIONS ABOUT THE SHOULDER

**Thoracic outlet syndrome** is often caused by compression of the lower brachial plexus and subclavian artery between the scalene muscles or by a cervical rib. It is associated with shoulder pain, which often radiates distally along the ulnar border of the forearm and hand. Pallor, coldness, and numbness, commonly of the ring and little fingers, may occur. The **Adson maneuver** is often positive: the ipsilateral radial pulse disappears when the patient abducts, extends, and externally rotates the shoulder while taking a deep breath with the head rotated maximally toward the affected side. Neurologic findings are subtle and affect both interosseous and hypothenar muscles, as well as cutaneous sensation of the little and ring fingers and the ulnar aspect of the forearm. Compression of the subclavian artery can be demonstrated by MRI-angiography.

**Acute brachial plexus neuritis** (acute brachial plexitis or brachial neuralgic amyotrophy) is an uncommon disorder characterized by a rapid onset of burning pain in the shoulder and upper arm, followed a few days later by profound upper-arm weakness affecting multiple muscles supplied by the upper brachial plexus: supraspinatus, infraspinatus, deltoid, and sometimes biceps. Diagnostic studies include electromyography (EMG) and MRI. The course of the neuritis is usually one of gradual recovery in 3 to 4 months.

**Quadrilateral space syndrome** is a rare disorder that results from compression of the axillary nerve and posterior circumflex humeral artery in the quadrilateral space. It is caused by athletic activities, GH dislocation, or shoulder surgery. Nondermatomal pain and paresthesia of the shoulder and upper posterior arm, exacerbated by abduction and external rotation, are the main symptoms. Tenderness over the quadrilateral space, aggravation of symptoms by external rotation, variable atrophy and weakness of the deltoid and teres minor muscles, and sometimes sensory loss over the anterolateral aspect of the shoulder and upper arm are the principal findings. The diagnosis can be confirmed by EMG, MRI, or MRI-angiography.

**Suprascapular nerve entrapment syndrome** is characterized by deep aching pain in the upper posterior aspect of the scapula, made worse by shoulder adduction, and by weakness of abduction and external rotation. It is caused by compression of the suprascapular nerve in the suprascapular notch, beneath the suprascapular or transverse scapular ligament, or by a ganglion or lipoma. It can also result from repetitive trauma due to excessive overhead movements. Local tenderness over the suprascapular notch and variable weakness and wasting of the supraspinatus and infraspinatus muscles are the main findings.

**Cervical radiculopathy,** caused by a cervical disk lesion, is associated with pain in the shoulder, radicular sensory symptoms, motor weakness, and reflex changes. Radicular pain and/or paresthesia may be reproduced by one of two tests. The **Spurling test** involves a combination of cervical spine extension and tilt toward the affected extremity with pressure applied downward on the patient's head. In the upper extremity root extension test, the patient's arm is extended, abducted, and externally rotated with the elbow and wrist extended, and the head is tilted to the opposite side. Diagnostic studies include cervical spine radiography, MRI, and nerve conduction studies.

## Physical Examination

### INSPECTION

With the patient sitting or standing and disrobed to the waist, both shoulders are inspected for symmetry, abrasions, scars, erythema, swelling, deformity, or muscle wasting. Subluxation of the AC joint is associated with a **step deformity,** with the acromion lying inferior to the clavicle. Swelling and prominence of the SC or AC joint may indicate arthritis or subluxation. Inferior subluxation of the GH joint is characterized by a positive **sulcus sign:** presence of a hollow, or sulcus, just below the acromion, made prominent by downward traction on the arm. Flattening of the rounded lateral aspect of the shoulder may indicate anterior dislocation of the GH joint or deltoid paralysis. Posterior dislocation of the GH joint is associated with flattening of the rounded anterior aspect of the shoulder.

Rupture of the long biceps tendon is associated with bunching up of the belly of the biceps muscle distally, made prominent by resisted elbow flexion and forearm supination (**Popeye sign** or **Popeye deformity**). In contrast, in a distal biceps tendon rupture, there is retraction of the muscle belly proximally. In thoracic scoliosis, one shoulder often appears lower than the other. **Sprengel deformity** is characterized by a congenitally small, high-riding scapula, sometimes associated with underdeveloped ipsilateral scapular muscles and webbing of the neck. **Winging of the scapula,** in which the medial border of the scapula moves away from the posterior chest wall, indicates injury to the long thoracic nerve with serratus anterior paralysis or other causes, such as clavicular malunion. Winging of the scapula is made more prominent by performance of a modified push-up against the wall with hands outstretched. Wasting of the supraspinatus muscle suggests a tear of the supraspinatus tendon or a suprascapular nerve lesion. Atrophy of the infraspinatus muscle can result from a tear of the infraspinatus tendon or a suprascapular nerve injury.

### PALPATION

Palpation should begin with assessment of all four shoulder articulations (sternoclavicular, acromioclavicular, glenohumeral, and scapulothoracic) for warmth, tenderness, swelling, crepitus, or masses. This will help localize the site of a patient's complaint and narrow the potential differential diagnosis.

Arthritis of the SC and AC joints is associated with local tenderness, synovial swelling, effusion, and sometimes crepitus on shoulder shrugging. Arthritis of the GH joint is characterized by global tenderness felt through the overlying deltoid in the anterior, lateral, and posterior subacromial areas.

Bicipital tenosynovitis is associated with localized tenderness over the tendon in the bicipital groove as the patient externally rotates the shoulder. The groove normally faces anteriorly when the shoulder is internally rotated 10°.

Scapulothoracic bursitis is associated with posterior subscapular pain and "grinding" or crepitus with scapulothoracic movements. In the so-called snapping scapula syndrome, protraction and retraction of the scapula is associated with audible and palpable grating, best felt at the superomedial corner of the scapula. This is caused by rubbing of the scapula over the underlying ribs.

### RANGE OF MOTION

Range-of-motion testing should include both active and passive assessments of shoulder forward flexion, extension, abduction, adduction, internal rotation, and external rotation. Limitations in active range of motion when passive range is maintained points to a deficit in the motor unit for that movement. This may be a problem with the motor nerve, muscle, or tendon responsible for the motion. Loss of passive range of motion is commonly associated with degenerative disorders, such as arthritis, or adhesive capsulitis.

Shoulder abduction involves synchronous movements of the GH, SC, and AC joints and rotation of the scapula on the chest wall. The initial 30° of abduction, achieved by contraction of the supraspinatus, takes place at the GH joint with little movement of the scapula. Beyond 30°, an approximate 2:1 ratio exists between GH and scapular movements. The combined movement is referred to as the *scapulohumeral rhythm.* Normal shoulder abduction is 180° (Figure 2-4).

To test forward flexion of the shoulder (deltoid, coracobrachialis, and biceps muscles; normal range 180°; Figure 2-5), the patient flexes the joint with the elbow extended, while the examiner stabilizes the scapula with one hand and resists forward flexion with the other hand placed over the upper arm. To test extension (latissimus dorsi, teres major, and deltoid muscles; normal range 60°; see Figure 2-5), the patient extends the shoulder, with the forearm fully pronated, while the examiner immobilizes the scapula and resists extension. With the shoulder abducted to 90° and the elbow flexed at 90°, the normal range of internal and external rotation is 90° each (Figure 2-6). With the elbow placed at the side at the waist, the normal range of external rotation is about 45° to 90°, and internal rotation is about 55° to 80° before its motion is stopped by the body; it may be as much as 120° if the patient can reach behind the back to touch the inferior angle of the opposite scapula (**Apley scratch test**). This is a functional movement required for daily activities, such as reaching a back pocket, scratching the back, or cleansing the perineum.

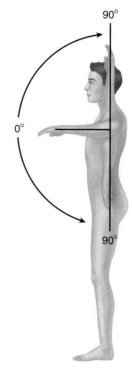

**FIGURE 2-6   SHOULDER INTERNAL AND EXTERNAL ROTATION.**

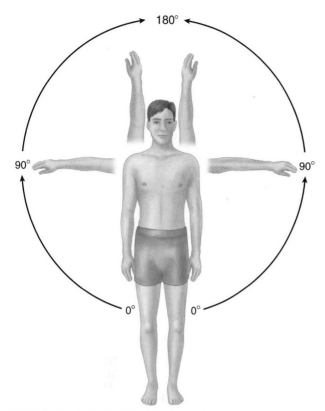

**FIGURE 2-4   SHOULDER ABDUCTION: SIDEWAYS ARC, CORONAL PLANE.**

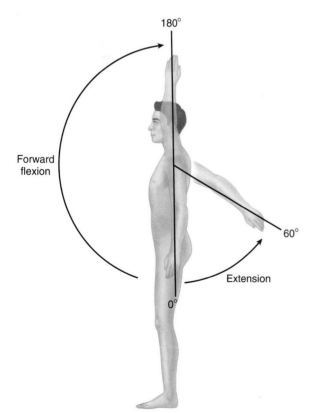

**FIGURE 2-5   SHOULDER FORWARD FLEXION AND EXTENSION.**

As the patient elevates the arm in abduction, the examiner can assess for the presence of a **painful arc.** Abduction to 45° to 60° is often painless. A painful arc between 60° and 120° is characteristic of subacromial impingement with rotator cuff tendinitis or subacromial bursitis. The pain often decreases beyond 120°, as the compression of the rotator cuff beneath the coracoacromial arch lessens. Pain between 120° and 180° may indicate abnormalities of the AC joint, whereas GH arthritis causes pain throughout the arc of abduction.

Reverse scapulohumeral rhythm, or greater scapulothoracic than GH movements during abduction, occurs in adhesive capsulitis; instead of the normal, smooth abduction, the patient appears to be "hitching" the entire shoulder complex upward. The capsular pattern of restricted shoulder movements typically observed in adhesive capsulitis is characterized by greater limitation of external rotation than of other movements. In GH arthritis, abduction and rotation are the earliest and most severely restricted movements.

## SPECIAL TESTS

Special tests for the shoulder are plentiful. These tests are designed to elicit evidence of impingement, rotator cuff dysfunction, superior labral anterior and posterior (SLAP) lesions, irritation of the long head of the biceps, and shoulder instability. The sensitivity and specificity of each of these tests has been an area of much study. A recent meta-analysis on this topic reveals significant variability in the sensitivity and specificity of these tests, depending on the population studied and the pretest probability of the condition in the population being studied. A summary of these findings is presented in Table 2-2.

| Special Test | Sensitivity (%) | Specificity (%) | N | Reference |
|---|---|---|---|---|
| Neer impingement sign | 86 | 49 | 552 | Park et al., 2005 |
| Hawkins impingement sign | 76 | 45 | 552 | Park et al., 2005 |
| Jobe sign, empty can sign | 53 | 82 | 552 | Park et al., 2005 |
| Lift-off test | 17 | 92 | 68 | Barth et al., 2006 |
| Belly press test | 40 | 98 | 68 | Barth et al., 2006 |
| Yergeson sign | 13 | 94 | 132 | Parentis et al., 2006 |
| Speed test | 40 | 75 | 552 | Park et al., 2005 |
| O'Brien test | 63 | 50 | 132 | Parentis et al., 2006 |
| Crank test | 13 | 83 | 132 | Parentis et al., 2006 |
| Anterior apprehension test | 72 | 96 | 363 | Farber et al., 2006 |
| Relocation test | 81 | 92 | 363 | Farber et al., 2006 |

**TABLE 2-2**

**SENSITIVITY AND SPECIFICITY OF COMMON SPECIAL TESTS OF THE SHOULDER**

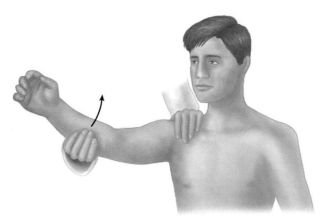

FIGURE 2-7   NEER IMPINGEMENT TEST.

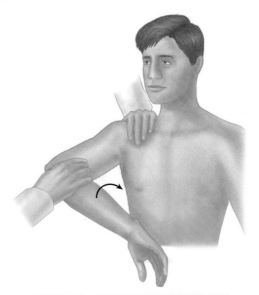

FIGURE 2-8   HAWKINS IMPINGEMENT SIGN.

### Tests for Shoulder Impingement

The **Neer impingement sign** is elicited with the patient seated and the examiner standing. Scapular rotation is prevented by one hand, as the other elevates the patient's arm midway between abduction and flexion. In a positive test, the patient experiences pain in the overhead position near the end of shoulder elevation, as the greater tuberosity impinges against the acromion (Figure 2-7). The pain can be relieved by subacromial injection of 5–10 mL of 1.0% lidocaine (Neer impingement test).

In the **Hawkins impingement sign,** the humerus is forward flexed to 90° and internally rotated, while the examiner's other hand restricts scapular movements (Figure 2-8). This causes impingement of the greater tuberosity against the anterior acromion with reproduction of the patient's symptoms. In patients with impingement and supraspinatus **tendinitis** or a tear, the **Jobe test, supraspinatus isolation test**, or **empty can sign** is positive: pain is elicited on resisted elevation of the arm to 90° midway between abduction and forward flexion, with the thumb pointing downward in internal rotation (Figure 2-9).

In subcoracoid impingement, there is impingement of the rotator cuff between the lesser tuberosity and the lateral aspect of the coracoid process during abduction and internal rotation. It commonly occurs in the throwing athlete. This type of impingement is associated with anteromedial shoulder pain and a positive **Gerber subcoracoid test:** painful restriction of internal rotation when the shoulder is abducted

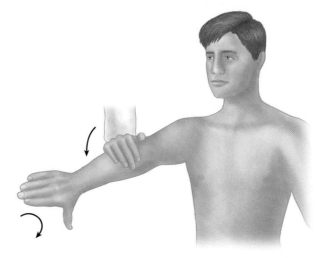

FIGURE 2-9   SUPRASPINATUS TEST (EMPTY CAN SIGN).

or flexed 90°, because this position produces the narrowest coracohumeral distance. Combined forward flexion, internal rotation, and cross-arm adduction (coracoid impingement test) also causes pain. The coracoid impingement test differs from the **O'Brien active compression test** for superior labral tears, in which the patient actively resists the examiner while performing the maneuver. The pain of subcoracoid impingement can be relieved by a lidocaine injection between the humeral head and the coracoid process.

### Tests of the Rotator Cuff

The supraspinatus (suprascapular nerve) is tested with the shoulder abducted 90°, flexed 30°, and internally rotated with the thumb pointing downward, while the examiner

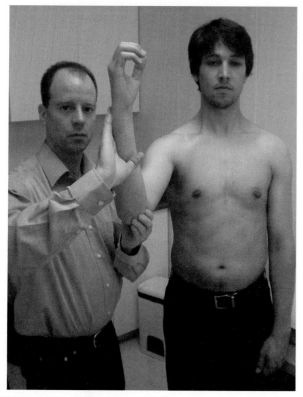

**FIGURE 2-10   HORNBLOWER TEST.** This test involves external rotation with the shoulder in 90° of abduction in the scapular plane. The elbow is flexed 90°, and the patient externally rotates against the resistance of the examiner's hand.

fixes the scapula with one hand and resists abduction with the other hand. This is known as the Jobe test, the supraspinatus isolation test, or the empty can sign (see Figure 2-9). In complete supraspinatus tears, the **drop-arm test** is positive: the patient is unable to actively maintain 90° of passive shoulder abduction or to slowly lower the arm to the side. With a partial supraspinatus tear, there is wasting and weakness of the supraspinatus muscle. The supraspinatus test, Neer impingement sign, and Hawkins impingement sign are often positive.

Infraspinatus and teres minor tears are associated with weakness of external rotation and a positive **external rotation lag sign (ERLS):** with the patient sitting, elbow 90° flexed, and the shoulder held by the examiner at 20° to 90° abduction and maximal external rotation, the patient is asked to actively maintain the position of external rotation as the examiner releases the wrist, and a "lag" or "angular drop" occurs. An alternative maneuver is the **Hornblower Test.** This test involves external rotation with the shoulder in 90° of abduction in the scapular plane. The elbow is flexed 90°, and the patient externally rotates against the resistance of the examiner's hand (Figure 2-10). Weakness of external rotation in this position constitutes a positive test.

Subscapularis tears are associated with weakness of internal rotation and a positive **subscapularis lift-off test:** after maximal internal rotation of the shoulder with the dorsum of the hand held against the inferior aspect of scapula, the patient is unable to lift the hand off his back (Figure 2-11). A subscapularis tear is also detected by the **belly press test** (Figure 2-12). The patient presses the abdomen with the palm of the hand (internal rotation), and if the subscapularis is intact, the patient can maintain pressure without the elbow dropping backward; if there is a subscapularis tear, maximal internal rotation cannot be maintained, and the elbow drops back behind the trunk (positive belly press test). The patient exerts pressure on the abdomen by extending the shoulder rather than by internally rotating it. The test is particularly useful in those patients with restricted internal rotation who cannot place the hand behind the back to perform the lift-off test.

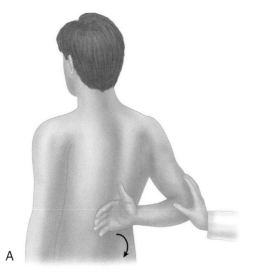

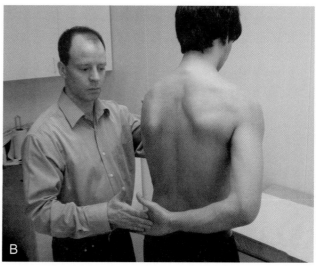

A          B

**FIGURE 2-11    LIFT-OFF TEST.**

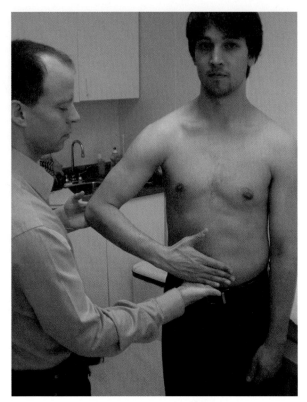

FIGURE 2-12    BELLY PRESS TEST.

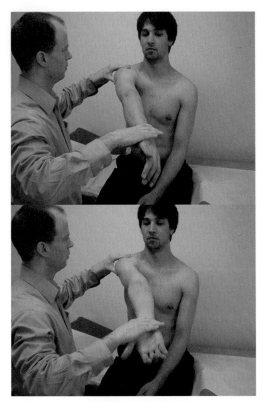

FIGURE 2-14    THE O'BRIEN ACTIVE COMPRESSION TEST.

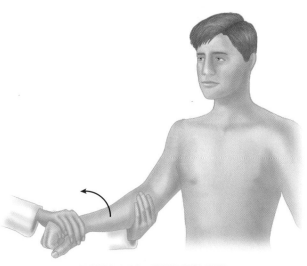

FIGURE 2-13    YERGESON SIGN.

### Tests for Labral Tears and Biceps Tendon Pathology

In bicipital tenosynovitis, pain in the bicipital groove is reproduced by resisted supination of the forearm with the elbow 90° flexed (**Yergeson sign** or **supination sign**; Figure 2-13) and by the more sensitive **Speed test,** in which there is pain on resisted flexion of the shoulder with the elbow extended and the forearm supinated.

In the **O'Brien active compression test,** with the patient standing, elbow extended, and the shoulder forward flexed 90°, adducted 15°, and internally rotated, so that the thumb points downward, the examiner applies downward pressure on the proximal forearm against the patient's resistance (Figure 2-14). The shoulder is then externally rotated, and the forearm is supinated, after which the maneuver is repeated. The test is positive if pain is elicited with the first maneuver but not with forearm supination. The thumb-down position (internal rotation) compresses the biceps–glenoid–labrum anchor, causing pain or a click deep in the shoulder if a SLAP lesion is present. In traumatic AC joint lesions, the O'Brien test may also produce more superficial pain on top of the shoulder.

Kim et al. (2001) described the **biceps load II test** to assess for the presence of a SLAP lesion. In this test, the patient lies supine with the arm abducted 120°, the elbow flexed to 90°, and the forearm supinated. The patient then flexes the elbow against the resistance of the examiner. Pain elicited by this maneuver constitutes a positive test.

The **crank test** is also used to detect a SLAP lesion. In this test the arm is abducted 160° with the elbow flexed 90°. The examiner then applies a compressive load across the joint while performing rotation of the shoulder. Pain, usually with external rotation of the shoulder, constitutes a positive test (Figure 2-15).

### Tests for Glenohumeral Instability

With the patient supine, the shoulder is 90° abducted and 90° externally rotated; the examiner then applies forward pressure to the posterior aspect of the humeral head (Figure 2-16A). In the presence of GH instability and recurrent anterior subluxation, the patient suddenly becomes apprehensive and complains of pain in the shoulder (positive anterior **apprehension test**). The **relocation test** or **containment**

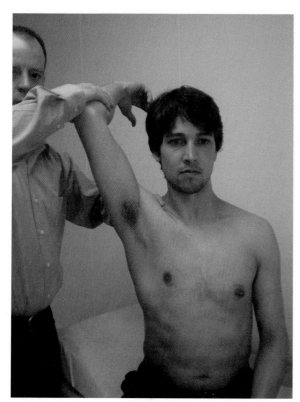

**FIGURE 2-15** **THE CRANK TEST.** This test is also used to detect a SLAP lesion.

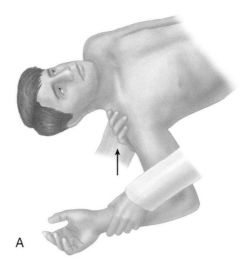

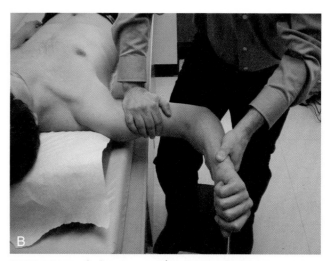

**FIGURE 2-16** **A,** Anterior apprehension test. **B,** Containment sign.

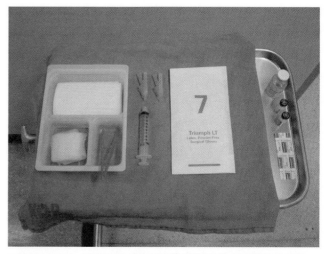

**FIGURE 2-17** **SOME REQUIRED EQUIPMENT FOR INJECTIONS AND ASPIRATIONS.**

**sign** (Figure 2-16B) is then performed by applying posterior pressure on the anterior aspect of the humeral head, to push the subluxed humeral head back in the glenoid fossa. Patients with GH instability and secondary impingement experience marked pain relief (positive **relocation test**). The examiner may then be able to externally rotate and extend the shoulder several degrees further while maintaining the posteriorly directed force on the humeral head. On release of the pressure on the humerus at this point, the patient complains of sudden pain (positive **anterior release sign**). The sign is more sensitive than the apprehension-relocation test in detecting occult GH instability.

With the patient standing or sitting and the arm at the side, the examiner stabilizes the scapula with one hand while drawing the humeral head anteriorly or posteriorly with the other hand. GH instability is associated with anterior and posterior displacement (translation) of the humeral head on the fixed scapula (positive **anterior** and **posterior drawer signs**). Laxity of the shoulder capsule and ligaments results in inferior subluxation of the humerus on downward traction of the arm, which produces a depression or hollow between the lateral edge of the acromion and the humeral head (positive **sulcus sign**).

## ASPIRATIONS AND INJECTIONS

Aspirations and injections are done about the shoulder for a number of indications. These include aspiration of a joint for synovial fluid analysis to aid in the diagnosis of inflammatory or septic arthritis. Injections of local anesthetic and antiinflammatory medications can be both diagnostic and therapeutic. Injection of a specific site, if accompanied by symptomatic relief, can help confirm the diagnosis and aid

further treatment. When performing these injections, sterile technique should always be adhered to. An example of the required equipment is shown in Figure 2-17.

For subacromial bursa and rotator cuff tendinitis, with the patient sitting and the shoulder slightly externally rotated, the

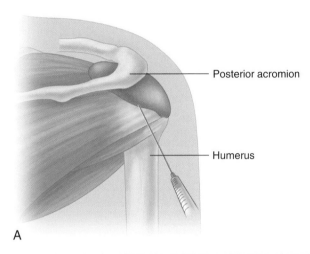

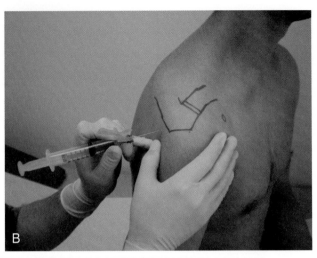

**FIGURE 2-18   INJECTION OF SUBACROMIAL BURSA AND ROTATOR CUFF TENDONS (POSTERIOR SUBACROMIAL APPROACH).**

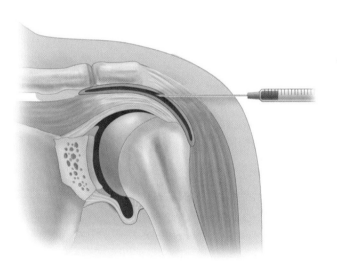

**FIGURE 2-19   ASPIRATION AND INJECTION OF SUBACROMIAL BURSA (LATERAL APPROACH).**

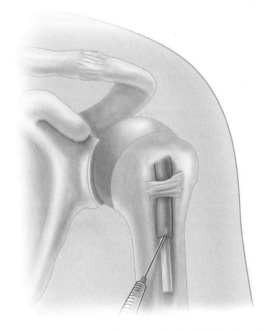

**FIGURE 2-21   INJECTION OF THE LONG BICEPS TENDON SHEATH.**

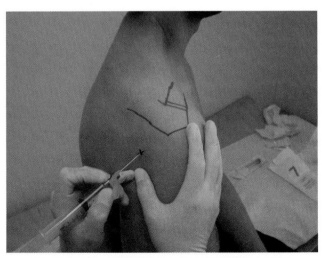

**FIGURE 2-20   INJECTION OF THE GLENOHUMERAL JOINT.**

needle is inserted about 1 cm below the posterior border of the acromion and directed medially, anteriorly, and slightly superiorly toward the tip of the coracoid process to a depth of 2 to 3 cm into the subacromial bursa (posterior subacromial approach, Figure 2-18). A fluid-distended subacromial bursa can be aspirated and injected via a lateral approach (Figure 2-19).

The GH joint is injected using a posterior approach. The entry point is two fingers' breadth medial and inferior to the palpated posterolateral border of the acromion. The needle is directed anteromedial toward the coracoid process (Figure 2-20).

For injection of the bicipital tendon sheath, the patient is sitting or supine, and the tendon is palpated in the bicipital groove while the shoulder is externally rotated. The point of maximum tenderness is marked, and the needle is inserted at an angle of 30° to 45° into the sheath. It is then directed superiorly along the tendon for about 2 cm before the sheath is aspirated and injected (Figure 2-21). Care is taken to avoid

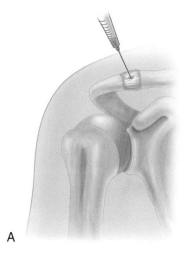
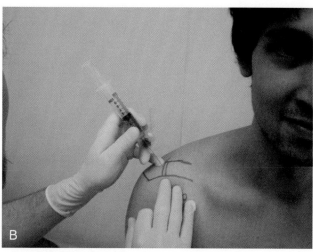

**FIGURE 2-22   INJECTION OF THE ACROMIOCLAVICULAR JOINT.**

intratendinous steroid injection, which can lead to tendon rupture.

The AC and SC joints are injected with the patient sitting or standing with the arm at the side. The AC or SC joint is palpated, and the needle is inserted via a superior and anterior approach into the joint and directed inferiorly to a depth of about 0.5 cm. Care is taken not to inject directly into the intraarticular disk, because this can damage the disk and cause secondary osteoarthritis (Figure 2-22).

## SELECTED READINGS

Almekinders, L.C., 2001. Impingement syndrome. Clin. Sports Med. 20, 491–504.

Barth, J.F., Burkhart, S.S., De Beer, J.F., 2006. The bear-hug test: A new and sensitive test for diagnosing a subscapularis tear. Arthroscopy 22, 1076–1084.

Debski, R.E., Parsons, I.M.I.V., Woo, S.L.-Y., Fu, F.H., 2001. Effect of capsular injury on acromioclavicular joint mechanics. J. Bone Joint Surg. Am. 83, 1344–1351.

Doukas, W.C., Speer, K.P., 2001. Anatomy, pathophysiology, and biomechanics of shoulder instability. Orthop. Clin. North Am. 32, 381–391.

Fam, A.G., 1998. Regional problems: The upper limbs in adults. In: Maddison, P.J., Isenberg, D.A., Woo, P., Glass, D.N. (Eds.), Oxford Textbook of Rheumatology, second ed. Oxford Medical Publications, Oxford, pp. 135–149.

Farber, A.J., Castillo, R., Clough, M., 2006. Clinical assessment of three common tests for traumatic anterior shoulder instability. J. Bone Joint Surg. 88 (A), 1467–1474.

Gerber, C., Krushell, R.J., 1991. Isolated rupture of the tendon of the subscapularis muscle. Clinical features in 16 cases. J. Bone Joint Surg. – British 73 (3), 389–394.

Gerber, C., Hersche, O., Farron, A., 1996. Isolated rupture of the subscapularis tendon. J. Bone Joint Surg. – American 78 (7), 1015–1023.

Hannafin, J.A., Chiaia, T.A., 2000. Adhesive capsulitis: A treatment approach. Clin. Orthop. 372, 95–109.

Hertel, R., Ballmer, F.T., Lombert, S.M., Gerber, C., 1996. Lag signs in the diagnosis of rotator cuff rupture. J. Shoulder Elbow Surg. 5 (4), 307–313.

Kim, S.H., Ha, K.I., Ahn, J.H., et al., 2001. Biceps load test II: A clinical test for SLAP lesions of the shoulder. Arthroscopy 17 (2), 160–164.

Lui, S.H., Henry, M.H., Nuccion, S.L., 1996. A prospective evaluation of a new physical examination in predicting glenoid labral tears. Am. J. Sports Med. 24 (6), 721–725.

Magee, D.J., 1987. The shoulder. In: Magee, D.J. (Ed.), Orthopedic Physical Assessment, first ed. WB Saunders, Philadelphia, pp. 62–91.

Neer II, C.S., 1983. Impingement lesions. Clin. Orthop. Rel. Res. 173, 70–77.

Neer II, C.S., Welsh, R.P., 1977. The shoulder in sports. Orthop. Clin. North Am. 8 (3), 583–591.

Neviaser, R.J., 1983. Painful conditions affecting the shoulder. Clin. Orthop. 173, 63–69.

Parentis, M.A., Glousman, R.E., Mohr, K.S., 2006. An evaluation for the provocative tests for the superior labral anterior posterior lesions. Am. J. Sports Med. 34, 265–268.

Park, H.B., Yokota, A., Gill, H.S., 2005. Diagnostic accuracy of clinical tests for the different degrees of subacromial impingement syndrome. J. Bone Joint Surg. 87 (A), 1446–1455.

Paulson, M.M., Watnik, N.F., Dines, D.M., 2001. Coracoid impingement syndrome, rotator interval reconstruction and biceps tenodesis in the overhead athlete. Orthop. Clin. North Am. 32, 485–493.

Rothman, R.H., Marvel Jr., J.P., Heppenstall, R.B., 1975. Anatomic considerations in the glenohumeral joint. Orthop. Clin. North Am. 6, 341–352.

Sarrafian, S., 1983. Gross and functional anatomy of the shoulder. Clin. Orthop. 173, 11–19.

Shaffer, B., Tibone, J.E., Kerlan, R.K., 1992. Frozen shoulder: A long-term follow-up. J. Bone Joint. Surg. Am. 74, 738–746.

Tallia, A.F., Cardone, D.A., 2003. Diagnostic and therapeutic injection of the shoulder region. Am. Fam. Physician 67, 1271–1278.

Tennet, T.D., Beach, W.R., Meyers, J.F., 2003. A review of the special tests associated with shoulder examination. Part I: The rotator cuff tests. Am. J. Sports Med. 31, 154–160.

Tennet, T.D., Beach, W.R., Meyers, J.F., 2003. A review of the special tests associated with shoulder examination. Part II: Laxity, instability, and superior labral anterior and posterior (SLAP) lesions. Am. J. Sports Med. 31, 301–307.

Williams, P.L., Warwick, R., Dyson, M., Bannister, L.H., 1989. Joints of the upper limb. Gray's Anatomy, thirty seventh ed. Churchill Livingstone, Edinburgh, pp. 499–516.

Yergason, R.M., 1931. Supination sign. J. Bone Joint Surg. – American 13 (1), 160.

# 3

# THE ELBOW

George V. Lawry • Elizabeth Grigoriadis

## Applied Anatomy

The elbow joint acts as both a hinge and a swivel, providing a stable link for lifting, pushing, or gripping and for positioning the hand in space. The hinge is formed by the humeroulnar (trochleoulnar) and humeroradial (capitelloradial) articulations at the cubital joint. The trochleoulnar is the principal joint, and the swivel is formed by the proximal radioulnar joint. These three joints share a common synovial cavity (Figure 3-1A).

Stability of the elbow depends upon congruity of the articulating bones, anterior capsule, ligaments, and surrounding muscles. The ulnar and radial collateral ligaments provide medial and lateral stability to the joint. The cup-shaped annular ligament encircles the radial head and holds it in the radial notch of the proximal ulna (Figure 3-2A, B).

The common flexor tendon of the elbow (pronator teres, flexor carpi radialis, palmaris longus, flexor digitorum superficialis, and flexor carpi ulnaris) takes origin from the medial epicondyle and supracondylar ridge of the humerus. The common extensor tendon (extensor carpi radialis longus and brevis, brachioradialis, extensor digitorum communis, extensor carpi ulnaris, and anconeus) originates from the lateral epicondyle, supracondylar ridge, and distal humerus. The biceps tendon crosses the elbow joint to insert into the radial tuberosity (see Figure 3-1B).

The ulnar nerve runs in a bony groove behind the medial epicondyle (the cubital tunnel; Figure 3-2A). The olecranon bursa, a subcutaneous cushion at the olecranon process, is synovially lined but is anatomically separate from the elbow joint (see Figure 3-2B).

Full elbow extension, the neutral (anatomic) position, is defined as 0° (not 180°). Some normal men, particularly muscular men, may lack 5° to 10° of full extension; normal women may demonstrate up to 10° of hyperextension.

With the elbow in full extension, there is normally a slight valgus angulation of the forearm with respect to the humerus. This angulation, referred to as the *carrying angle,* is due to the oblique shape of the trochlea (see Figure 3-1A) and is normally ~5° to 10° in men and ~10° to 25° in women (Figure 3-3). This angle allows the forearms to clear the hips during the normal arm swing of ambulation and is important for carrying objects at the side, without requiring shoulder abduction. Excessive deviation of the forearm away from the body is referred to as *cubitus valgus,* and deviation of the forearm toward the body is called *cubitus varus.*

Normal elbow flexion is from 0° to 160°. Any deficit in full extension is referred to as a *flexion contracture* (joint contracture in the direction of flexion). The brachialis, biceps, and brachioradialis are the primary flexors of the elbow, and the large, powerful triceps and small, relatively weak anconeus are the extensors. A minimum total arc of elbow flexion–extension of ~100° is required for normal activities.

Pronation of the forearm and hand (palm of hand facing posteriorly in anatomic position) and supination (palm facing anteriorly in anatomic position) occur at the proximal and distal radioulnar joints, as the radial head pivots on the capitellum while the distal radius rotates around the distal ulna (see Figure 3-3). Normal pronation is ~75° and supination is ~85°. The pronator teres and pronator quadratus are the principal pronators, and the biceps and supinator muscles are the primary supinators of the radioulnar joints. A minimum total arc of pronation–supination of ~100° is required for normal activities.

## History

Elbow pain is commonly caused by a relatively small number of conditions that include periarticular (tendinitis and bursitis), articular (arthritis), bone (fracture and dislocation), or neurologic problems (Table 3-1).

Evaluation of elbow pain focuses on answering three important questions: 1) Is there evidence of major trauma or injury? 2) Can symptoms and signs be adequately explained by a local problem confined to the elbow? 3) Is there evidence of a more generalized articular process, of which the elbow is only a part, or a neurologic process with elbow symptoms referred from another site?

Assessment of elbow pain requires a careful delineation of pain characteristics and associated features. A helpful mnemonic for characterizing pain in almost any site is OPQRST: O = onset, P = precipitating (and ameliorating) factors, Q = quality, R = radiation, S = severity, and T = timing.

An initial screening history should readily identify those patients with elbow pain secondary to fracture or dislocation, and an appropriate radiographic and orthopedic assessment can be initiated. A history of unusually intense or repetitive recreational or occupational activity is important, particularly in patients with suspected tendinitis. Furthermore, pain characteristics may suggest neurologic involvement (burning, tingling, and radiation), and associated symptoms in the neck and shoulder or wrist and hand may suggest pain

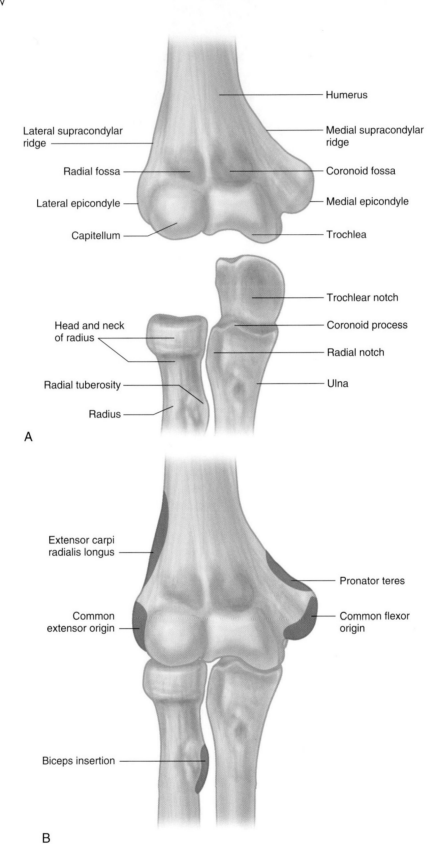

Humerus

Lateral supracondylar ridge

Medial supracondylar ridge

Radial fossa

Coronoid fossa

Lateral epicondyle

Medial epicondyle

Capitellum

Trochlea

Trochlear notch

Head and neck of radius

Coronoid process

Radial notch

Radial tuberosity

Ulna

Radius

A

Extensor carpi radialis longus

Pronator teres

Common extensor origin

Common flexor origin

Biceps insertion

B

**FIGURE 3-1    A & B, BONES AND MUSCLES OF THE ELBOW.**

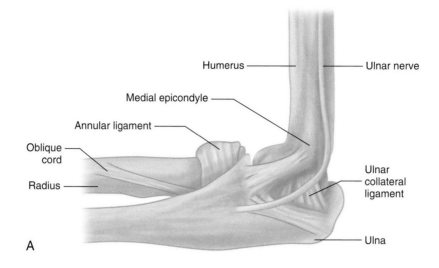

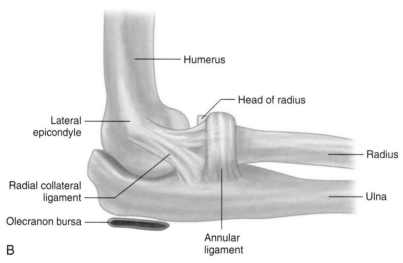

**FIGURE 3-2    A & B, LIGAMENTS OF THE ELBOW.**

referral from a site other than the elbow. Additional articular symptoms in other sites may suggest a more generalized process, such as rheumatoid or psoriatic arthritis.

## Physical Examination

### INSPECTION

With the elbows in full extension, observe the carrying angle, noting any valgus or varus angulation. Inspect the elbow for erythema (acute inflammation or infection) or any vesicular rash, such as Herpes zoster. Check the extensor surface of the elbow for any subcutaneous nodules (rheumatoid nodules or gouty tophi) or cutaneous psoriasis (psoriatic arthritis). Inspect the olecranon for any visible swelling (olecranon bursitis; Table 3-2).

### PALPATION

Slide your other hand along the forearm to the olecranon surface. Note any palpable subcutaneous nodules or swelling of the olecranon bursa. Swelling of the olecranon bursa

presents itself as visible and/or palpable distension directly overlying the olecranon, often looking like the comic character Popeye (Figure 3-4).

Next, identify the small depression normally present between the olecranon and the lateral epicondyle, which is especially visible during full extension (Figure 3-5). This depression is the first area to be obliterated by an elbow effusion. Now, use your examining thumb to identify and palpate the lateral epicondyle. Slide your thumb slightly distally while you gently pronate and supinate the forearm with your other hand still in the "handshake" position. You can now feel the patient's radial head, moving under your palpating thumb. The joint space between the lateral epicondyle and radial head should now be readily appreciable with only skin and subcutaneous tissue between your thumb and the joint line itself. Next, continue palpating the joint line while you bring the elbow into full extension. Note whether there is any pain or resistance to full extension, frequently seen with elbow joint synovitis (Figure 3-6).

Swelling of the elbow joint results in progressive obliteration of the normal small lateral sulcus and a "boggy" or thickened feel to the usually well-defined depression (joint line) between the lateral epicondyle and radial head.

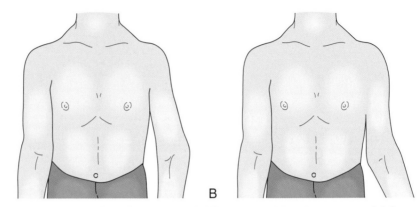

**FIGURE 3-3   CARRYING ANGLE. A,** Right arm: normal; left arm: varus. **B,** Right arm: normal; left arm: valgus.

| TABLE 3-1 |
|---|
| **COMMON CAUSES OF ELBOW PAIN** |
| **Periarticular** |
| Olecranon bursitis |
| *Lateral epicondylitis (tennis elbow)* |
| *Medial epicondylitis (golfer's elbow)* |
| **Articular** |
| Arthritis: crystalline (gout and pseudogout), rheumatoid, psoriatic; osteoarthritis (secondary); septic |
| Trauma: dislocation |
| **Osseous** |
| Trauma: fracture |
| **Neurologic** |
| Cubital tunnel syndrome (ulnar nerve) |
| Radiculopathy (referred pain due to cervical disk lesion) |

| TABLE 3-2 |
|---|
| **EXAMINATION OF THE ELBOW** |
| **Basic Exam** |
| **INSPECTION** |
| ____ Note carrying angle |
| ____ Inspect elbow (rashes, abrasions, or skin breaks) |
| **PALPATION** |
| ____ Palpate olecranon surface (subcutaneous nodules, tophi) |
| ____ Palpate olecranon bursa (bursal swelling; nodules, tophi) |
| ____ Palpate lateral joint line (synovial swelling) |
| **RANGE OF MOTION** |
| ____ Assess elbow flexion |
| ____ Assess elbow extension |
| ____ Check forearm pronation and supination |
| **SPECIAL TESTING: LATERAL EPICONDYLITIS** |
| ____ Palpate lateral epicondyle and ~1 cm distally |
| ____ Test resisted wrist extension |
| **SPECIAL TESTING: MEDIAL EPICONDYLITIS** |
| ____ Palpate medial epicondyle and ~1 cm distally |
| ____ Test resisted wrist flexion and forearm pronation |
| **SPECIAL TESTING: ULNAR NEUROPATHY** |
| ____ Palpate nerve in ulnar groove |
| ____ Check Tinel sign |
| ____ Palpate for snapping ulnar nerve |
| ____ Test forced elbow flexion (~60 seconds) |
| ____ Inspect interosseous muscles and assess strength of fifth finger to resisted abduction |
| ____ Check sensation in fourth and fifth fingers |
| **SPECIAL TESTING: LIGAMENTOUS LAXITY** |
| ____ Stress medial and lateral collateral ligaments |

Furthermore, synovial distension may produce a visible or palpable bulge when the elbow is moved into full extension, as intraarticular pressure increases.

If your examining thumb strays laterally, sliding off the lateral epicondyle toward the olecranon, you may find a soft swelling in normal individuals that may feel very much like synovitis, but it is not: you have just discovered the belly of the anconeus muscle. (Keeping your examining thumb in contact with the lateral epicondyle at all times when palpating the lateral joint line will prevent this error.)

Palpable swelling, most frequently combined with the patient's hesitation to permit full elbow extension due to pain, confirms the presence of synovial swelling and/or fluid within the elbow joint.

## RANGE OF MOTION

Next, flex and extend each elbow. Full elbow flexion places the proximal forearm against the distal biceps (~150° to 160°). Elbow extension returns the joint to the outstretched anatomical position (0°). Place your hand under the olecranon to assist you in detecting any deficit in full extension (flexion contracture). Return the elbow to 90° of flexion and assess forearm pronation and supination.

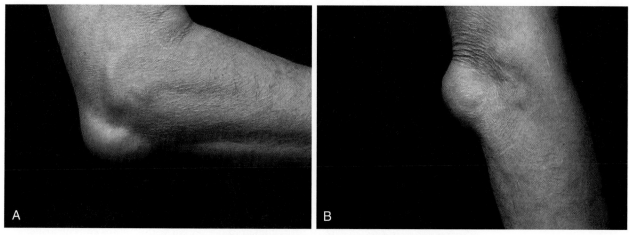

**FIGURE 3-4    SWOLLEN OLECRANON BURSA IN FLEXION AND EXTENSION.**

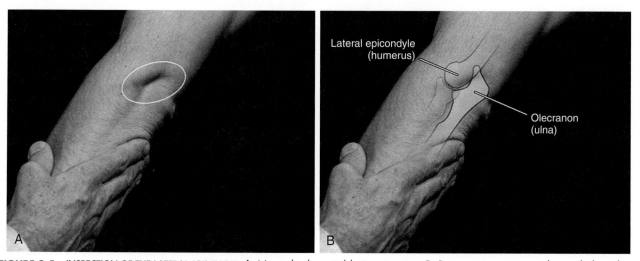

**FIGURE 3-5    INSPECTION OF THE LATERAL JOINT LINE. A,** Normal sulcus visible in extension. **B,** Bony anatomy present beneath the sulcus.

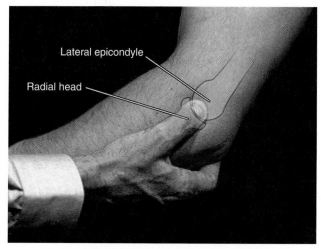

**FIGURE 3-6    PALPATION OF THE LATERAL JOINT LINE.**

## SPECIAL TESTING

Next, if appropriate, assess for the presence of **lateral epicondylitis** ("tennis elbow"). Bring the elbow into partial flexion and identify the lateral epicondyle with your thumb. Palpate the lateral epicondyle and apply progressively increasing

pressure to the epicondyle itself. Then, move ~1 cm distally and again apply pressure. Note any focal tenderness. Next, place the elbow in full extension and support the forearm with your arm. Ask the patient to make a fist and "cock it back" (fingers flexed and wrist extended). Supply downward force against the dorsum of the hand against the patient's resistance. Note any lateral elbow pain (Figure 3-7).

Similarly, if appropriate, assess for the presence of **medial epicondylitis** ("golfer's elbow"). Bring the elbow into partial flexion and identify the medial epicondyle with your thumb. Palpate the medial epicondyle and apply progressively increasing pressure to the epicondyle itself. Then, move ~1 cm distally and again apply pressure. Note any focal tenderness. Next, ask the patient to extend the elbow with the palm down, forearm in pronation. Then, ask them to flex the wrist (fingers extended and wrist flexed). Supply force against the palmar surface, attempting to move the wrist back to neutral while they resist. Note any medial elbow pain.

If indicated, assess for **ulnar nerve irritation or compression** in the cubital tunnel. Palpate the ulnar nerve at the medial aspect of the elbow, in the ulnar groove. Tap lightly over the ulnar nerve (Tinel sign, Figure 3-8) and note any pain or tingling radiating to the forearm and lateral hand (fourth and fifth digits). Next, palpate the ulnar groove

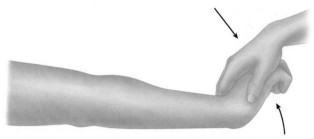

**FIGURE 3-7    LATERAL EPICONDYLITIS: RESISTED WRIST EXTENSION TEST.**

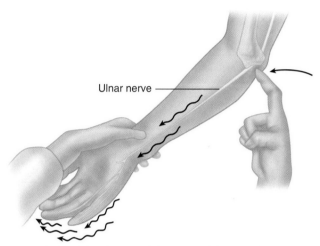

Ulnar nerve

**FIGURE 3-8    CUBITAL TUNNEL SYNDROME: TINEL SIGN.**

during elbow flexion and extension. Note whether the nerve slips in and out of the ulnar groove. Finally, move the elbow into full flexion for ~60 seconds. Note any tingling or numbness in the ulnar aspect of the hand. Complete your assessment by checking for interosseous wasting and abduction strength of the fifth finger. Check sensory function over the fourth and fifth fingers. Note any deficits.

In patients with suspected **ligamentous instability,** assess ulnar and radial ligamentous integrity with the elbow in 10° to 20° of flexion to unlock the olecranon process from its fossa. With the humerus stabilized with one hand, apply an abduction (valgus) force to the distal forearm to assess the medial (ulnar) collateral ligament, and apply an adduction (varus) force to the distal forearm to assess the lateral (radial) collateral ligament.

## Common Disorders of the Elbow

### SKIN AND SUBCUTANEOUS ABNORMALITIES

The extensor surface of the elbow is one of the most common sites for **rheumatoid nodules.** They may be firm to hard subperiosteal swellings on the olecranon extensor surface or several centimeter-sized rubbery, moveable nodules in the olecranon bursa. The bursa itself is the most common site of **tophi** in patients with gout. Early tophi may be barely noticeable to your examining fingers but later may be present as rubbery, moveable nodules indistinguishable from rheumatoid nodules.

The extensor surface of the elbow is one of the most common sites of **cutaneous psoriasis.** Musculoskeletal complaints in patients with psoriasis raise the question of whether the patient might have psoriatic arthritis.

### OLECRANON BURSITIS

The olecranon bursa is one of the few bursae where irritation and inflammation present as clinically visible and palpable swelling (Figure 3-4). **Acute trauma** may lead to hemorrhagic swelling within the bursa. **Repetitive pressure** on the olecranon may cause chronic swelling. The two most common inflammatory conditions affecting the olecranon bursa are **rheumatoid arthritis** and **gout.** The bursa may swell suddenly and painfully in acute gout; may swell gradually with minimal pain, warmth, or erythema in rheumatoid arthritis; or may swell imperceptibly over time with the development of rheumatoid nodules or gouty, tophaceous deposits.

The most clinically urgent problem involving the bursa is **septic olecranon bursitis.** Signs of significant acute inflammation usually develop over hours to days. It is very important to check for abrasions, scabs, or broken skin anywhere from the fingers to the elbow in all patients with olecranon bursitis, as these findings may be the only clue that leads you to appropriately suspect septic bursitis. Septic bursitis typically occurs in otherwise healthy adult men engaged in physical work involving frequent trauma to the forearms and elbows (e.g., plumbers, gardeners, and construction workers). *Staphylococcus aureus* is the most common pathogen.

Septic olecranon bursitis frequently has significant accompanying features of cellulitis with widespread erythema, subcutaneous swelling, and edema. Rapid bursal swelling due to bacterial infection may lead to bursal disruption with obliteration of normal anatomic landmarks around the entire elbow, leading to concern over the more serious possibility of septic arthritis.

Several historical and physical examination features are very helpful in differentiating septic bursitis from arthritis. First, carefully assess the time course and progression of swelling. Frequently the patient will recall Popeye-like swelling initially, indicating olecranon bursitis as the underlying problem. Second, patients with septic arthritis will usually have severe pain with limited elbow flexion and extension. Range of motion is surprisingly preserved in patients with septic-cellulitic olecranon bursitis. Gentle, passive elbow extension is perhaps the most useful discriminating maneuver to help differentiate between these two possibilities. Finding intense inflammation with intact elbow extension focuses attention on the olecranon bursa. Intense inflammation with incomplete, painful elbow extension directs attention to the joint itself.

### ELBOW JOINT SWELLING

Elbow joint swelling in the context of acute injury or major trauma should prompt a comprehensive orthopedic evaluation for fracture or dislocation, which is beyond the scope of this discussion. The elbow joint is not often a site of primary osteoarthritis but is a site of secondary osteoarthritis related to prior significant injury or repetitive trauma. Inflammatory processes involving the elbow include crystalline arthritis (gout or pseudogout), rheumatoid arthritis, psoriatic arthritis, or infection (bacterial and rarely tuberculous or fungal infections).

Elbow joint swelling is usually experienced by the patient as a deep, poorly localized ache aggravated by motion, especially at the extremes of flexion and extension. The greater the acuteness of inflammation, the more likely the patient is to hold the elbow at ~70° of flexion, the position of lowest intraarticular pressure. Chronic elbow synovitis, as in rheumatoid arthritis, may be minimally tender or not tender at all, with no accompanying warmth or visible erythema; acute inflammatory synovitis, as in acute crystalline arthritis, may exhibit all the cardinal features of inflammation. If the elbow joint is the site of an acute inflammatory monoarthritis, it is imperative, as with all acute monoarthritides, to aspirate the joint to check for crystals or infection.

## LATERAL EPICONDYLITIS

Patients with lateral epicondylitis, also called **tennis elbow,** usually complain of localized pain and tenderness at the lateral epicondyle, often accompanied by a mild aching discomfort in the proximal forearm. Contrary to its common name, "tennis elbow" it is usually vocational, recreational, or idiopathic in origin and rarely due to playing tennis. Understanding that lateral epicondylitis is not primarily an elbow problem, but related to use of the wrist and hand, helps greatly in understanding the problem. The extensor carpi radialis is a powerful extensor of the wrist and is essential to an important hand function, the power grip. To firmly grasp objects with the hand, the finger flexor tendons must be stretched to allow the flexor muscles in the forearm to exert maximal force. It is "setting the wrist up" (in extension) in preparation for a power grip that results in the generation of significant force at the proximal tendon and its insertion site.

Patients with lateral epicondylitis usually have an insidious onset of pain over weeks to months. On careful questioning, most will associate lifting heavy objects (milk cartons, hammers, suitcases) with increased pain. On occasion, actions as simple as shaking hands will provoke symptoms. Some patients will be concerned that they are "losing hand strength."

Localized tenderness is present just distal, medial, and slightly anterior to the lateral epicondyle, over the common extensor tendon, particularly that part derived from the extensor carpi radialis brevis muscle. The pain is increased by resisted dorsiflexion of the wrist with the elbow in extension.

## MEDIAL EPICONDYLITIS

Medial epicondylitis, or so-called **golfer's elbow,** is far less common than lateral epicondylitis. Like tennis elbow, it also is not primarily an elbow problem; it relates instead to an overuse syndrome from repetitive strain of the common flexor tendon involved in both forearm pronation and wrist flexion. Insertional tendinitis at the medial epicondyle may result from swimming, baseball pitching, or golfing. It is often associated with aching discomfort in the medial epicondyle and flexor aspect of the proximal forearm. It is increased by lifting, grasping, and other activities that require frequent wrist flexion and forearm pronation. There is tenderness at and just distal to the medial epicondyle over the origin of the common flexor tendon, particularly that portion derived from the pronator teres and flexor carpi radialis muscles. Resisted pronation of the forearm and resisted flexion of the wrist with the elbow in full extension are clinically helpful provocative maneuvers. Flexion of the fingers, rather than of the wrists, may sometimes elicit pain at the medial

epicondyle. In addition, it is important to examine the ulnar nerve in the cubital tunnel, as ulnar neuropathy may also cause medial elbow pain.

## ULNAR ENTRAPMENT NEUROPATHY

Cubital tunnel syndrome is due to entrapment of the ulnar nerve in its groove behind the medial epicondyle. It is characterized by medial elbow pain, paresthesia along the ulnar aspect of the forearm into the ring and little fingers, and sometimes a weak hand grip with fatigue and clumsiness. Tenderness is often present over the ulnar nerve, and the Tinel sign is usually positive. Atrophy of the hypothenar muscles may be present.

Causative mechanisms include sudden direct trauma to the ulnar nerve in the ulnar groove, repetitive injury to the nerve from chronic pressure on hard surfaces, such as desks and countertops, and repetitive stretching injury of the nerve in its groove due to occupational or sport activities involving prolonged elbow flexion such as skiing, throwing, and racquet sports. Chronic progressive entrapment of the nerve may also be due to scarring or bony osteophyte formation as a result of remote major trauma to the elbow (fracture or dislocation).

# Aspiration and Injection of the Elbow

## OLECRANON BURSA

Using a retracted ballpoint pen, mark the skin on the ulnar surface ~1 cm distal to the olecranon bursa. Prep the skin with iodine solution and allow to air dry, then prep with alcohol. Using a 22 gauge needle, inject 1% or 2% lidocaine subcutaneously at the site of your skin mark and advance proximally into the bursa. Use an 18 gauge needle on a 10 mL syringe for aspiration. While you advance the needle with your dominant hand, use your nondominant hand to squeeze the bursa between your gloved thumb and index fingers to help guide the needle into the bursa. Occasionally, the bursal fluid is loculated, and you will need to make a series of passes with the needle to aspirate fluid (your nondominant hand is invaluable here in helping stabilize and center the bursa). Aspirate the bursal fluid. If clinically appropriate, inject corticosteroid (Figure 3-9). This

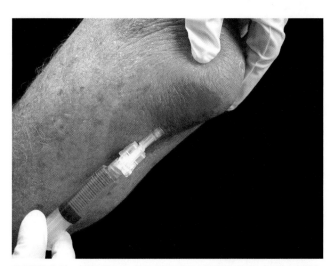

**FIGURE 3-9** ASPIRATION AND INJECTION OF THE OLECRANON BURSA.

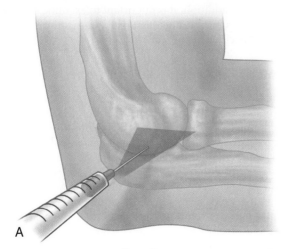

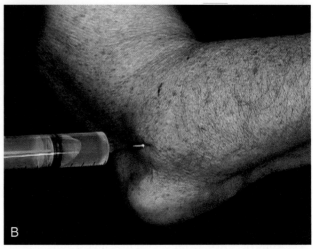

**FIGURE 3-10  A,** Approach to elbow joint aspiration and injection. **B,** Rheumatoid patient with joint effusion being aspirated at lateral joint line (plus nodules in the anatomically separate olecranon bursa).

subcutaneous "tunnel" technique avoids puncturing the bursa on its exposed extensor surface and decreases the likelihood of fluid leakage with elbow flexion subsequent to aspiration.

### Elbow Joint

With the elbow in ~45° of flexion, identify the lateral epicondyle, the radial head, and the tip of the olecranon. These three points form a triangle, the center of which is the entry point for the lateral approach to the elbow joint. Palpate at the center of this imaginary triangle, and use a retracted ballpoint pen to make a mark at this site. Prep the skin with iodine and allow to air dry, then prep with alcohol. Use a 22 gauge needle and 1% or 2% lidocaine to create a skin wheel. Now, direct the needle along a plane parallel to an imaginary line connecting the lateral and medial epicondyles. (Using this angle of needle entry, rather than perpendicular to the skin surface, may make successful aspiration much easier; Figure 3-10A). As you advance the needle, inject lidocaine until you enter the joint space. Once in the joint space, change syringes and aspirate with a 10 mL syringe. Occasionally, the synovial fluid is loculated and may be difficult to aspirate initially. You may need to rotate the needle or make several small changes in needle depth to obtain fluid (gentle, rather than forceful, suction is often the most effective). Aspirate the joint completely if possible. If clinically appropriate, inject corticosteroid.

### Lateral Epicondyle

Using a retracted ballpoint pen, mark the skin at the point of maximum tenderness, usually ~1 cm distal to the lateral epicondyle (Figure 3-11). Prep the skin with iodine and allow to air-dry, then prep with alcohol. Using a 25 gauge needle, inject 1% or 2% lidocaine into the skin. Advance into and through the extensor tendon and inject additional lidocaine. Leave the needle in place, exchange syringes, and inject a corticosteroid preparation. After completing the procedure, it is useful to repeat resisted elbow extension. If the injection has been appropriately placed, there should be a dramatic decrease in pain with this provocative maneuver, frequently surprising the patient.

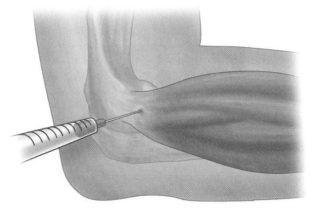

**FIGURE 3-11    INJECTION TECHNIQUE FOR LATERAL EPICONDYLITIS.**

The technique is similar for injecting the medial epicondyle. Inject directly on or just distal to the epicondyle. Avoid injecting posterior to the epicondyle in the region of the ulnar groove and ulnar nerve.

### SELECTED READINGS

Allander, E., 1974. Prevalence, Incidence and Remission Rates of Common Rheumatic Diseases and Syndromes. Scand. J. Rheumatol. 3, 145–153.

Binder, A.I., Hazleman, B.L., 1983. Lateral Humeral Epicondylitis: A Study of Natural History and the Effect of Conservative Therapy. Br. J. Rheumatol. 22, 73–76.

Buehler, M.J., Thayer, D.T., 1988. The Elbow Flexion Test: A Clinical Test for the Cubital Tunnel Syndrome. Clin. Orthop. 233, 213–216.

Canoso, J.J., Barza, M., 1993. Soft Tissue Infections. Clin. Rheum. Dis. 19, 293–309.

Kraushaar, B.S., Nirschl, R.P., 1999. Tendinosis of the Elbow (tennis elbow). J. Bone Joint Surg. Am. 81, 259–278.

Magee, D.J., 2002. Orthopedic Physical Assessment, fourth ed. Saunders, Philadelphia, PA.

Regan, W.D., Morrey, B.F., 1993. The Physical Examination of the Elbow. In: Morrey, B.F. (Ed.), The Elbow and Its Disorders, WB Saunders, Philadelphia, PA.

Yocum, L.A., 1989. The Diagnosis and Non-operative Treatment of Elbow Problems in the Athlete. Clin. Sports Med. 8, 439–451.

# 4

# THE WRIST AND HAND

Arthur A. M. Bookman • Herbert P. von Schroeder • Adel G. Fam

## Applied Anatomy

### THE HAND (Fam, 2003)

The hand is the chief sensory organ of touch and is uniquely adapted for grasping. The radial side of the hand performs a **pinch grip** between the fingers and thumb, and the ulnar side performs a **power grip** between the fingers and palm. The bones of the hand can be divided into a central, fixed unit for stability and three mobile units for dexterity and power. The fixed unit consists of the eight carpal bones tightly bound to the second and third metacarpals (Figure 4-1). The three mobile units projecting from the fixed unit are:

- The thumb—the first carpometacarpal (CMC) joint permits extension, flexion, abduction, and adduction for powerful pinch and grasp and fine manipulations
- The index finger, endowed with independent extrinsic extensors and flexors and powerful intrinsic muscles—for precise movements alone or with the thumb
- The middle, ring, and littlew fingers—for power grip, a function enhanced by slight movements of the fourth and fifth metacarpals at their CMC articulations

The axis of the wrist and hand is an extension of the longitudinal axis of the radius and the third metacarpal, with the wrist in the neutral position. Because of the changing position of the wrist and hand with forearm pronation and supination, it is best to describe locations in the wrist awnd hand as volar (palmar), dorsal, radial, and ulnar rather than anterior, posterior, lateral, and medial. The hand has two arches: a *longitudinal arch,* in the mid palm from wrist to fingers, and a *transverse arch* across the mid palm. In the resting position, the fingers are normally slightly flexed at the metacarpophalangeal (MCP) and interphalangeal (IP) joints; this is referred to as the **resting flexion cascade of the fingers.**

### WRIST JOINT

The radiocarpal joint is the proximal articulation of the wrist and is an ellipsoid joint between the distal radius and articular disk proximally and the scaphoid, lunate, and triquetrum distally (see Figure 4-1). The capsule is strengthened by the **radiocarpal (dorsal and volar) ligaments.** The articular disk, or **triangular fibrocartilage** of the wrist, joins the radius to the ulna. Its base is attached to the ulnar border of the distal radius, and its apex is attached to the root of the ulnar styloid process. The synovial cavity of the distal radioulnar joint is L-shaped and extends distally beneath the triangular fibrocartilage but is usually separated from the radiocarpal joint.

The radiocarpal, midcarpal distal radioulnar, and CMC joints do not communicate under normal circumstances. The presence of any communication, tested by wrist arthrography or MR arthrograms, implies torn ligaments or a torn capsule between them. The midcarpal joint is in continuity with the intercarpal joints except for the pisotriquetral articulation, which communicates with the radiocarpal joint (see Figure 4-1).

The carpal bones form a volar concave arch or **carpal tunnel,** with the pisiform and hook of the hamate on the ulnar side and the scaphoid tubercle and the crest of the trapezium on the radial side. The four bony prominences are joined by the **flexor retinaculum (transverse carpal ligament),** which forms the roof of the carpal tunnel. The distal flexion crease of the wrist marks the proximal border of the retinaculum. The **palmaris longus** (absent in 10% to 15% of the population) partly inserts into the flexor retinaculum and partly fans out into the palm, forming the **palmar aponeurosis (fascia).** The aponeurosis broadens distally and divides into four digital slips that attach to the finger flexor tendon sheath, MCP joint capsules, and proximal phalanges. There is usually no digital slip to the thumb (Markison, 1987).

Twenty-four extrinsic tendons cross the wrist and provide a unique combination of power and dexterity to the hand. Each tendon is enclosed for part of its course in a **tenosynovial sheath.** A wrist or finger tendon sheath is lined by an inner or **visceral synovial layer** that adheres closely to the tendon and an outer or **parietal synovium** that covers the inside of the fibrous tendon sheath. The visceral and parietal synovial tubes are united longitudinally by the **mesotendon,** a synovial fold that transmits vessels and nerves to the tendon. The mesotendon may disappear partially in some tendon sheaths and may be represented by threads or **vinculae.**

The **common flexor tendon sheath** encloses the long flexor tendons of the fingers (Strauch, 1985) (flexor digitorum superficialis and flexor digitorum profundus) and extends from approximately 2.5 cm proximal to the wrist crease to the mid palm. It runs with the flexor pollicis longus tendon sheath and the median nerve through the carpal tunnel (Figure 4-2). The tendon sheath of the little finger is usually continuous with the common flexor sheath. The **flexor pollicis longus tendon** to the thumb runs through a separate tenosynovial sheath but may join the common

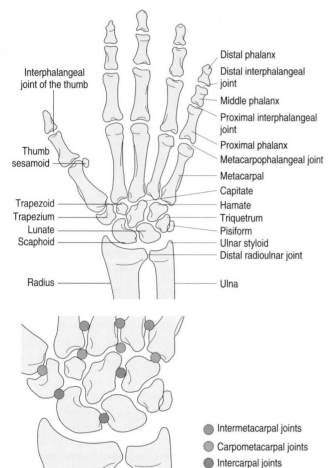

Interphalangeal joint of the thumb

Distal phalanx
Distal interphalangeal joint
Middle phalanx
Proximal interphalangeal joint
Proximal phalanx
Metacarpophalangeal joint
Metacarpal
Capitate
Hamate
Triquetrum
Pisiform
Ulnar styloid
Distal radioulnar joint

Thumb sesamoid

Trapezoid
Trapezium
Lunate
Scaphoid

Radius

Ulna

● Intermetacarpal joints
● Carpometacarpal joints
● Intercarpal joints

**FIGURE 4-1    BONES AND JOINTS OF THE WRIST AND HAND.** (From Hochberg H, Silman AJ, Smolen JS, et al., eds.: *Rheumatology,* 3rd ed. London: Mosby, 2003.)

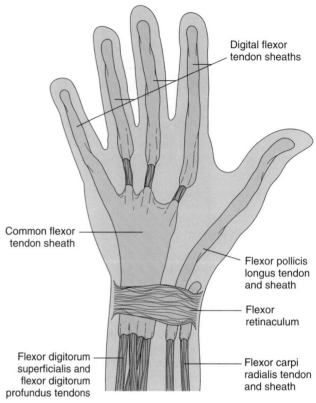

Digital flexor tendon sheaths

Common flexor tendon sheath

Flexor pollicis longus tendon and sheath

Flexor retinaculum

Flexor digitorum superficialis and flexor digitorum profundus tendons

Flexor carpi radialis tendon and sheath

**FIGURE 4-2    FLEXOR TENDONS AND TENDON SHEATHS OF THE WRIST AND FINGERS.** (From Hochberg H, Silman AJ, Smolen JS, et al., eds.: *Rheumatology,* 3rd ed. London: Mosby, 2003.)

flexor sheath. The **flexor carpi radialis** is invested in its own short tendon sheath as it crosses the volar aspect of the wrist between the split radial attachment of the flexor retinaculum. It is separated from the carpal tunnel by the deep portion of the transverse carpal ligament. The flexor retinaculum straps down the flexor tendons as they cross at the wrist. The ulnar nerve, artery, and vein cross over the retinaculum but are covered by a fibrous band, the superficial part of the transverse carpal ligament, to form the ulnar tunnel, or **Guyon canal.**

On the dorsum of the wrist, the extensor tendons pass through six tenosynovial, fibro-osseous tunnels beneath the **extensor retinaculum:** 1) the abductor pollicis longus and extensor pollicis brevis (usually in a single sheath), which constitute the first, most radial extensor compartment; 2) the extensor carpi radialis longus and brevis; 3) the extensor pollicis longus; 4) the extensor digitorum communis and extensor indicis proprius; 5) the extensor digiti minimi; and 6) the extensor carpi ulnaris, the most ulnar extensor compartment (Figure 4-3). Each tenosynovial sheath extends about 2.5 cm proximally and distally from the retinaculum. The extensor retinaculum, by its deep attachments to the distal radius and ulna, binds down and prevents

bowstringing of the extensor tendons as they cross the wrist. The **anatomic snuffbox** corresponds to the depression between the extensor pollicis longus tendon and the tendons of the abductor pollicis longus and extensor pollicis brevis.

Movements of the wrist include flexion (in the volar direction), extension, ulnar deviation, radial deviation, and circumduction. The intercarpal joints, particularly the lunate-capitate joint, contribute to wrist extension and flexion. Prime wrist flexors are the flexor carpi radialis, flexor carpi ulnaris, and palmaris longus. The prime extensors are the extensor carpi radialis longus and brevis and extensor carpi ulnaris.

## CARPOMETACARPAL JOINTS

The first CMC joint is a saddle-shaped, very mobile articulation between the trapezium and the base of the first metacarpal. It allows 40° to 50° of thumb flexion–extension parallel to the plane of the palm and 40° to 70° of adduction–abduction perpendicular to the plane of the palm. These movements are important in bringing the thumb in opposition with the fingers. The second and third CMC joints are relatively fixed, but the fourth and fifth are mobile, allowing the fourth and fifth metacarpals to flex forward (15° to 30°) toward the thumb during power grip.

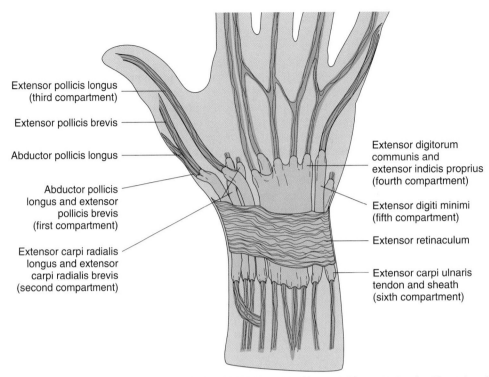

**FIGURE 4-3**    **EXTENSOR TENDONS AND TENDON SHEATHS OF THE WRIST.** (From Hochberg H, Silman AJ, Smolen JS, et al., eds.: *Rheumatology*, 3rd ed. London: Mosby, 2003.)

## METACARPOPHALANGEAL JOINTS

The metacarpophalangeal (MCP) joints are ellipsoid joints that lie about 1 cm distal to the knuckles (metacarpal heads; see Figure 4-1). Their capsule is strengthened by the **radial and ulnar collateral ligaments** on the sides and by the **volar plate** on the volar surface. Because of the cam shape of the metacarpal head, the collateral ligaments are loose in the neutral position, allowing radial and ulnar deviations, but become tight in the flexed position, preventing side-to-side motion, referred to as a **sagittal cam effect.** The **deep transverse metacarpal ligament** joins the volar plates of the second to fifth MCP joints. The MCP joint of the thumb is large and has two sesamoid bones overlying its volar surface.

When the long extensor tendon of the digit reaches the metacarpal head, it is joined by the tendons of the interossei and lumbricals and expands over the dorsum of the MCP joint and digit to form the **extensor hood** or **extensor expansion** (Figure 4-4). The expansion divides over the dorsum of the proximal phalanx into an intermediate slip, inserted principally into the base of the middle phalanx, and two collateral slips inserted into the base of the distal phalanx (von Schroeder, 1997).

The first MCP joint permits 50° to 70° flexion and 10° to 30° extension. Radial and ulnar deviations are limited to less than 10° to 20°. The other MCP joints allow 100° flexion, 10 to 20° extension, and 35° of radial and ulnar movement. The extensor pollicis brevis, extensor indicis proprius, extensor digitorum communis, and extensor digiti minimi extend the MCP joints (von Schroeder, 1993). The flexors are the flexor pollicis brevis, lumbricals, interossei, and flexor digiti minimi brevis, assisted by the

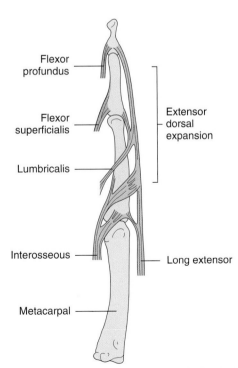

**FIGURE 4-4    TENDON INSERTIONS OF THE FINGER AND EXTENSOR DORSAL EXPANSION (HOOD).** (From Hochberg H, Silman AJ, Smolen JS, et al., eds.: *Rheumatology*, 3rd ed. London: Mosby, 2003.)

long flexors. Radial and ulnar movements at the second to fifth MCP joints are a function of the intrinsic muscles.

## INTERPHALANGEAL JOINTS

The proximal interphalangeal (PIP) and distal interphalangeal (DIP) joints of the fingers and the IP joint of the thumb are hinge joints. Their capsules are strengthened by the collateral ligaments on the sides and by the volar plates on the volar surface, which serve to limit hyperextension, particularly at the PIP joints. Unlike the MCP joints, the radial and ulnar collateral ligaments remain taut in all positions, providing side-to-side stability throughout the range of movement.

The **flexor tendon sheaths for the fingers** enclose the tendons of the flexor digitorum superficialis and profundus to their insertions on the middle and distal phalanges, respectively. The sheaths extend from just proximal to the MCP joints to the bases of the distal phalanges (see Figure 4-2). The flexor sheath of the little finger is often continuous with the wrist common flexor tendon sheath. The **thumb flexor pollicis longus tendon sheath** extends proximally to the carpal tunnel. Segmental condensations, or **annular pulleys,** in the digital flexor sheaths prevent bowstringing of

the tendons and are biomechanically critical for full digital flexion.

The PIP joints can hyperextend by 10° in young adults, and the joints allow 100° to 120° volar flexion. The DIP joints permit 50° to 80° volar flexion and 5° to 10° extension. The IP joint of the thumb allows 80° to 90° volar flexion and 20° to 35° extension. The flexor digitorum superficialis flexes the PIP joints, and the flexor digitorum profundus flexes the DIP joints of the fingers. The prime extensors are the interossei and the lumbrical muscles. The flexor pollicis longus flexes the IP joint of the thumb, and the extensor pollicis longus extends the joint.

# Differential Diagnosis of Wrist and Hand Pain

Pain in the wrist and hand may have its origin in the bones and joints of the wrist and hand, palmar fascia, tendon sheaths, nerve roots, peripheral nerves, or vascular structures, or it may be referred from the cervical spine, thoracic outlet, shoulder, or elbow (Table 4-1). Important points in

| TABLE 4-1 | |
|---|---|
| **DIFFERENTIAL DIAGNOSIS OF WRIST AND HAND PAIN** | |
| **Articular** | Arthritis of wrist, MCP, PIP, and/or DIP joints |
| | Joint neoplasms |
| **Periarticular** | |
| Subcutaneous | RA nodules, gouty tophi, glomus tumor |
| Palmar fascia | Dupuytren contracture |
| Tendon sheath | de Quervain tenosynovitis |
| | Wrist volar flexor tenosynovitis (including carpal tunnel syndrome) |
| | Thumb or finger flexor tenosynovitis (trigger thumb or finger) |
| | Pigmented villonodular tenosynovitis |
| Acute calcific periarthritis | Wrist, MCP, and rarely PIP and DIP |
| | Ganglion |
| **Osseous** | |
| | Fractures, neoplasms, infection |
| | Osteonecrosis including Kienböck disease (lunate) and Preiser disease (scaphoid) |
| **Neurologic** | |
| *Nerve entrapment syndromes* | |
| Median nerve | Carpal tunnel syndrome (at wrist) |
| | Pronator teres syndrome (at pronator teres) |
| | Anterior interosseous nerve syndrome |
| Ulnar nerve | Cubital tunnel syndrome (at elbow) |
| | Guyon canal (at wrist) |
| Radial nerve | Radial nerve palsy, radial tunnel syndrome, Wartenberg syndrome |
| Lower brachial plexus | Thoracic outlet syndrome, Pancoast tumor |
| Cervical nerve roots | Herniated cervical disk, tumors |
| Spinal cord lesion | Spinal tumors, syringomyelia |
| **Vascular** | |
| Vasospastic disorders (Raynaud disease) | Scleroderma, occupational vibration syndrome |
| Vasculitis with digital ischemic ulcers | SLE, RA |
| **Referred Pain** | |
| Cervical spine disorders | |
| Chronic regional pain syndrome | Shoulder–hand syndrome, causalgia, reflex sympathetic dystrophy |
| **Cardiac** | |
| Angina pectoris | |

DIP, distal interphalangeal; MCP, metacarpophalangeal; PIP, proximal interphalangeal; RA, rheumatoid arthritis; SLE, systemic lupus erythematosus

the history include onset, location, character, duration, and modulating factors of pain. A history of unaccustomed, repetitive, or excessive hand activity is particularly important in the diagnosis of wrist, thumb, or finger tenosynovitis caused by an overuse syndrome. A detailed occupational history is essential for determining whether the hand tendinitis is work related, either as a cumulative trauma disorder or as an acute injury. Abnormal tensile stresses that exceed the elastic limits of tendons can lead to cumulative microfailure of the molecular links between tendon fibrils, a phenomenon referred to as *fibrillar creep*. With aging, tendons become less flexible and less elastic, rendering them more susceptible to injury. A shortened musculotendinous unit, from lack of regular stretching exercises, is more prone to cumulative trauma disorder (Strauch, 1985).

## Physical Examination of the Hand and Wrist

### INSPECTION

With the hands on the examining table, one makes a general assessment of age, inflammation, atrophy, deformity, and asymmetry. Age-related changes include prominent veins on the dorsum of the hand, mild atrophy of the intrinsic muscles, lentigines on the skin and osteoarthritic prominences at the CMC joint at the base of the thumb, and osteophytes at the DIP and PIP joints. Osteoarthritic changes are ubiquitous and eventually result in such enlargement of the small joints of the fingers and deformity (McMurtry, 1986).

Acute inflammation following trauma is characterized by regional swelling and erythema. In contrast, chronic inflammation has less swelling and erythema and is often associated with synovitis of the joints and/or tendons. Deformity of any or all joints occurs with all forms of arthritis, but the particular pattern of deformity can be characteristic of a specific type of arthritis and will aid in diagnosis. The deformity will mirror the patient's functional limitations and will dictate treatment. Assessing the deformity, motion, and instability of each digit requires a systematic approach and thorough documentation. Detailed wrist palpation, including provocative testing for carpal instability, will allow the examiner to localize specific disorders.

## Physical Examination of the Digits

The fingers are inspected for swelling of the MCP, PIP, or DIP joints, deformities, clubbing, subcutaneous nodules, gouty tophi, age-related osteoarthritic Heberden or Bouchard nodes, sclerodactyly, telangiectasia, ischemic digital ulcers, pitted scars, nail fold infarcts, periungual erythema, or psoriatic lesions of the skin or nails.

To test for stability of the MCP joints of the fingers, each joint is individually flexed to 90° to tighten the radial and ulnar collateral ligaments, and the corresponding metacarpal is then held in one hand while the other hand moves the finger, held at the proximal phalanx, from side to side to test the integrity of the collateral ligaments. For the thumb MCP joint, the joint is flexed to 30° to neutralize the stabilizing effects of the adductor and extensor muscles, while

the joint is tested in ulnar and radial deviation and compared to the opposite side. Injury of the ulnar collateral ligament of the first MCP joint is associated with tenderness over the ligament and swelling of the joint ("skier's thumb" or "gamekeeper's thumb"). The stability of the radial and ulnar collateral ligaments of the PIP and DIP joints can be assessed by applying side strain with the joint in the neutral position.

### ASSESSING SYNOVITIS OF THE JOINTS AND TENDONS

Chronic synovitis is best assessed on the dorsum of the hand and wrist, where the tendons and joints are close to the surface and have fewer constraining structures over them. Synovitis of the joints produces a diffuse swelling over the joint and is uniformly tense and sometimes warm to the touch (McMurtry, 1986). The PIP and DIP joints are palpated by compressing laterally and/or gently forcing the joint into hyperextension for tenderness (stress pain). Synovial thickening and effusion are assessed by the examiner using the thumbs and forefingers of both hands placed on opposite sides of the joint (Figure 4-5). An effusion can be detected by the balloon sign: compression of the joint by one hand produces ballooning, or a hydraulic lift, sensed by the other hand. Unlike PIP synovitis, dorsal knuckle pads produce a nontender thickening of the skin localized to the dorsal surface of the PIP joints. The thumb MCP joint can be assessed in the same way. Tenderness in the MCP joints of the second to fifth digits are assessed by placing the examiner's thumb under the volar aspect of the proximal phalanx, the fingers on the dorsum of the hand, and stressing the joint into hyperextension. An effusion can be ballooned by compressing the flexed MCP joint from the dorsoradial side and palpating the fluctuance from the dorsoulnar side (Figure 4-6).

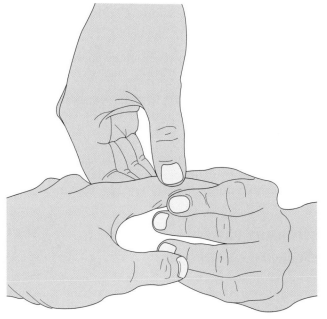

**FIGURE 4-5  PALPATION OF THE PROXIMAL INTERPHALANGEAL JOINT.** (From Hochberg H, Silman AJ, Smolen JS, et al., eds.: *Rheumatology*, 3rd ed. London: Mosby, 2003.)

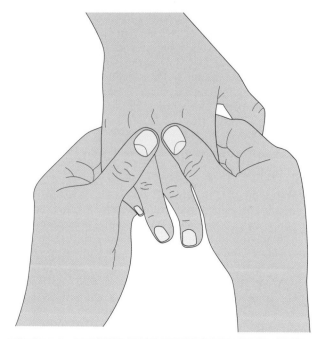

**FIGURE 4-6  PALPATION OF THE METACARPOPHALANGEAL JOINT.** (From Hochberg H, Silman AJ, Smolen JS, et al., eds.: *Rheumatology*, 3rd ed. London: Mosby, 2003.)

Tenosynovial effusion of the extensor tendons is localized to the tendon sheath and may have an hourglass configuration as it expands on either side of the extensor retinaculum. When the fingers are actively extended, the distal margin of the swelling moves proximally and folds in, like a sheet being tucked under a mattress (**tuck sign**). The swelling may be more oval over the extensor carpi ulnaris. Chronic synovial effusions of the tendons may have a gel-like consistency with minimal erythema. Synovitis of the wrist is best appreciated by placement of the examiner's thumbs side by side transversely across the carpus, just distal to the Lister tubercle. Pressure on the wrist by one thumb causes the other to be lifted by fluid or soft-tissue swelling.

Finger flexor tenosynovitis produces linear tenderness, volar swelling, thickening, nodules, and/or crepitus of the tendon sheath (sausage finger). Trigger fingers are tested by palpation for nodules, tenderness, clicking, or catching at each flexor A1 pulley at the distal palmar crease. Flexion contractures of the PIP or DIP joints of the fingers can be due to tendon or intrinsic muscle contractures. Relaxing these structures by flexing the MCP joints while attempting to extend the PIP or DIP joints will determine whether the contracture is articular or due to extrinsic structures.

## DEFORMITY PATTERNS

### Rheumatoid Arthritis (RA)

RA can result in deformity of any or all of the joints of the hand and wrist. Boutonnière's deformity describes a finger with flexion of the PIP joint and hyperextension of the DIP joint (Figure 4-7A). A swan-neck deformity describes the appearance of a finger in which there is hyperextension of the PIP joint and flexion of the DIP joint (see Figure 4-7B).

In swan-neck finger deformity, tightness and shortening of the intrinsic muscles (interossei and lumbricals) results in restriction of PIP flexion when the MCP joint is extended. Therefore, with the MCP joint extended, the range of PIP flexion is less than when the MCP joint is flexed (positive Bunnell test). Z-shaped deformity of the thumb is caused by flexion of the MCP joint and hyperextension of the IP joint (see Figure 4-7C). Z-shaped deformities, finger deformities, and MCP synovitis produce a diffuse swelling of the joint that may obscure the valleys between the knuckles. MCP joint deformities include ulnar drift, volar subluxation (often visible as a "step"), and flexion deformities. The extensor tendons subluxate into the valleys on the ulnar side of their respective digits.

Wrist deformities are common in RA and include volar subluxation of the carpus with a visible step opposite the radiocarpal joint, carpal collapse (loss of carpal height, the distance from distal radius to base of metacarpal, to less than half the length of the third metacarpal), and radial posturing (radial deviation) of the carpus. Chronic arthritis of the distal radioulnar joint results in instability and dorsal subluxation of the ulnar head with "piano key" movements on upward or downward pressure.

### Juvenile Rheumatoid Arthritis (JRA)

Children with inflammatory arthritis develop growth retardation of the metacarpals leading to shortening of one or several digits. Inflammation at the wrist results in lost range of motion, in large measure due to fusion of the capitate to the bones that surround it.

### Psoriatic Arthritis

Telescoped shortening of the digits, produced by partial resorption of the phalanges, occurs with psoriatic arthritis or sometimes with RA. It is often associated with concentric wrinkling of the skin (opera-glass hand), and psoriatic lesions of the skin or nails can occur. Fused IP joints are also common.

### Dupuytren Contracture

In Dupuytren contracture, the aponeurotic thickening of the palmar fascia may extend distally to involve the digits. The fingers become flexed at the MCP joints by taut fibrous bands, or "cords," that radiate from the palmar fascia, and the hand cannot be placed flat on a table (positive tabletop test) (Saar, 2000).

### Post-traumatic Deformities

Mallet finger is a flexed DIP joint with no active extension due to an acute or chronic rupture of the terminal tendon of the extensor mechanism. A *dropped knuckle* refers to fracture of the metacarpal shaft proximal to the MCP joint, with disappearance of the prominence of the metacarpal head typically involving the fifth metacarpal "boxer's fracture." Fracture and malunion of the distal radius, such as a Colles fracture, is associated with dorsal displacement of the distal fragment and a "silver" or "dinner fork" deformity.

### Osteoarthritis (OA)

Osteophytes at the DIP and PIP joints (Heberden and Bouchard nodes respectively) occur with age or following trauma and may be associated with gradual ulnar drift of the

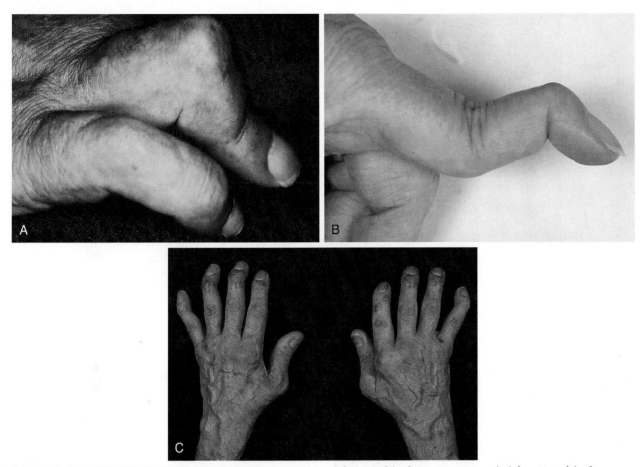

**FIGURE 4-7   DEFORMITIES OF THE FINGER AND THUMB. A,** Boutonnière's deformity of the finger. **B,** swan-neck deformities of the fingers. **C,** Z-shaped deformities of the thumbs. (From Hochberg H, Silman AJ, Smolen JS, et al., eds.: *Rheumatology,* 3rd ed. London: Mosby, 2003.)

fingers. "Squaring" of the carpometacarpal (CMC) joint at the base of the thumb due to OA is particularly common. The thumb eventually becomes more adducted toward the hand. At the wrist, OA can result in chronic swelling, bland effusions, and decreased active and passive range of motion.

### Other Deformity Patterns

Congenital anomalies of the hand and wrist can be the clue to diagnoses such as Albright disease or arthrogryposis (De Smet, 2002).

## PALPATION OF THE WRIST: ASSESSING BONES, JOINTS, AND LIGAMENTS

The wrist is best examined in the "arm wrestling" position, with the patient's elbow on the examining table and the hand up (Figure 4-8). In this position, motion in all directions is checked, all of the carpal bones can be palpated, and key ligaments can be assessed. The scaphoid (Beckenbaugh, 1984) is palpated at three points (Figure 4-9). First, the scaphoid tubercle is prominent on the volar aspect of the wrist proximal to the thenar eminence (Figure 4-9A). It becomes more prominent as the scaphoid flexes in the volar direction while the wrist is brought into radial deviation. The Watson maneuver (scaphoid shift) (Watson, 1988) tests the integrity of the scapholunate ligament (see Scapholunate Ligament, p. 39; Figure 4-19). Tenderness directly at the scaphoid tubercle may be due to a fracture of the tubercle or osteoarthritis at the scaphotrapeziotrapezoid (STT) joint. The

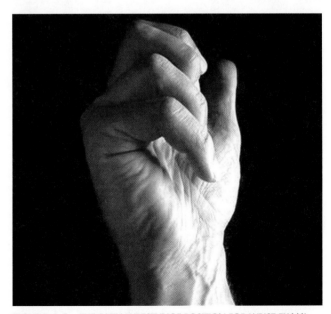

**FIGURE 4-8   THE "ARM WRESTLING" POSITION FOR WRIST EXAMINATION.** The wrist is best examined in this position, with the patient's elbow on the examining table and the hand up. This allows the patient to relax their hand and allows the examiner to easily maneuver the wrist, palpate all of the carpal bones, and test for stability.

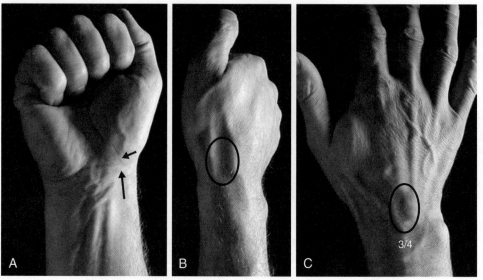

**FIGURE 4-9    THREE POINTS FOR PALPATING THE SCAPHOID. A,** The scaphoid tubercle (arrows) becomes more prominent as the scaphoid flexes during wrist movement into radial deviation. **B,** The scaphoid waist is palpable in the anatomical snuffbox (circle), between the extensor tendons of the first compartment and the EPL; the scaphoid ridge becomes more prominent here with ulnar deviation of the wrist. **C,** The proximal portion of the scaphoid is palpable in the soft spot (circle) between the tendons of the third and fourth (3/4) compartment, just distal to the Lister tubercle.

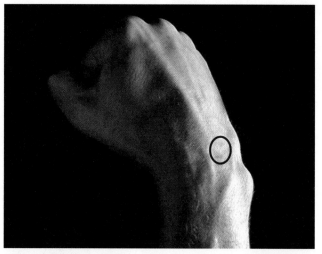

**FIGURE 4-10    THE LUNATE (CIRCLE) IS PALPATED JUST BEYOND THE DISTAL RADIOULNAR JOINT.**

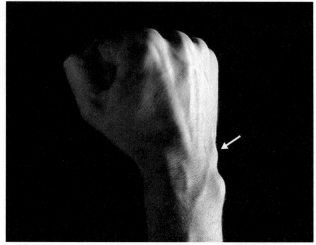

**FIGURE 4-11    THE DORSAL PROMINENCE OF THE TRIQUETRUM (ARROW).** This point is readily palpable distal to the head of the ulna. it becomes more prominent with radial deviation.

second point to palpate the scaphoid is the anatomical snuffbox on the radial aspect of the wrist (Figure 4-9B). With the examiner's fingertip in the snuffbox, ulnar deviation of the wrist will allow palpation of the scaphoid ridge in the waist of the bone. Tenderness here represents acute fracture (De Smet, 2002), fracture nonunion (pseudoarthrosis), or synovitis. The third place to examine the scaphoid and scapholunate region is between the third and forth compartments on the dorsum of the wrist and about 2 cm distal to the Lister tubercle (Figure 4-9C). This "soft spot" is also used for injecting the radiocarpal joint and as an arthroscopic portal. Palpations at this spot during wrist flexion will bring the proximal portion of the scaphoid under the examiner's finger.

The lunate is directly distal to the distal radioulnar joint, below the tendons of the fourth and fifth compartments (Figure 4-10). It is not readily distinguishable, but like the proximal scaphoid, the lunate is palpable as the wrist is

brought into full flexion. Tenderness here is associated with Kienböck osteonecrosis of the lunate.

The dorsal prominence of the triquetrum is readily palpable distal to the ulnar head (Figure 4-11). It becomes more prominent in radial deviation. Tenderness may be associated with a shear fracture of the prominence resulting from a fall. A smaller prominence may be palpable on the ulnar side of the triquetrum. Volar to the triquetrum is the pisiform at the base of the hypothenar eminence (Figure 4-12); a sesamoid bone in the flexor carpi ulnaris tendon, it is slightly mobile in a radial-ulnar direction. Osteoarthritis may develop at the synovial joint between the pisiform and triquetrum and is characterized by pain on direct palpation of the joint at the ulnar side of the hand and by pushing the pisiform against the triquetrum while moving it side to side.

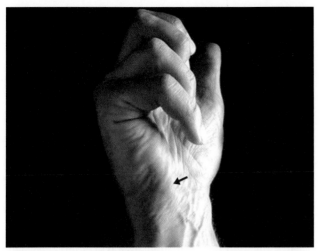

**FIGURE 4-12    THE PISIFORM (ARROW).** Located at the base of the hypothenar eminence, it can be mobilized a few millimeters in the radial and ulnar direction.

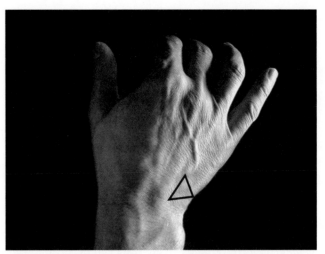

**FIGURE 4-14    THE DORSUM OF THE HAMATE.** A flat region (triangle) just distal to the dorsal triquetral prominence.

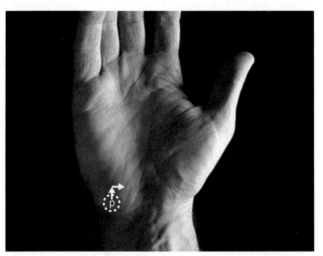

**FIGURE 4-13    THE HOOK OF THE HAMATE.** A vague prominence just distal and radial from the pisiform (p).

Approximately 2 cm distal and radial to the pisiform is the hook of the hamate (Figure 4-13). It is a vaguely defined prominence on palpation and may be slightly tender in normal individuals. It is significantly tender following a fracture or fracture nonunion of the hook. The dorsum of the hamate is palpable as a flat region just distal to the dorsal triquetral prominence (Figure 4-14). The fifth carpometacarpal (CMC) joint is assessed by palpating directly over the joint as the metacarpal is flexed and extended. Tenderness may represent post-traumatic or *de novo* osteoarthritis at the joint.

The dorsum of the capitate is palpable at its waist (Figure 4-15). This is a soft spot at the base of the third metacarpal. It is located approximately 1 cm distal and ulnar to the dorsal soft spot, where the scaphoid was palpated just beyond the Lister tubercle.

The dorsal base of the index metacarpal flares, and this bony prominence can increase with age and osteoarthritis, in which case it is referred to as a *carpal boss* (Figure 4-16). The trapezoid bone is located proximal to the prominent base of the second metacarpal and under the extensor carpi radialis longus tendon that inserts into the metacarpal.

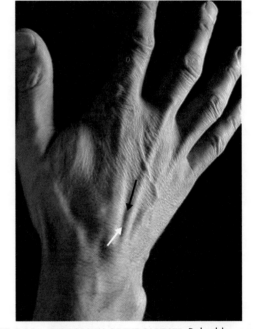

**FIGURE 4-15    THE DORSUM OF THE CAPITATE.** Palpable as a soft spot at the base of the third metacarpal (black arrow) and distal to the soft spot of the proximal scaphoid (white arrow).

At the base of the thumb metacarpal, and with rotational movement of the metacarpal, the CMC joint and the trapezium are palpated (Figure 4-17). This is best assessed by pinching the joint region on either side of the tendons of the first compartment with the pulps of the examiner's index finger and thumb. Osteoarthritis is particularly common at this joint, especially in women, and can be assessed by axially loading the metacarpal and translocating or "grinding" the CMC joint to look for pain and crepitus. "Squaring" of the joint is noted on inspection of patients with moderate to severe osteoarthritis.

The distal radioulnar joint (DRUJ) is palpable as a sulcus on the radial side of the ulnar head on the dorsum of the wrist. It is a forearm joint through which pronation and supination occur. This arc of motion is tested with the elbow locked on the examination table, or with the elbow at the patient's side, to prevent shoulder contribution to the motion. Tenderness at the joint is most commonly due to post-traumatic osteoarthritis due to fracture, incongruence associated with a distal radius fracture or malunion; *de novo* osteoarthritis and inflammatory arthritis, especially rheumatoid, occur here as well.

The sulcus between the ulnar head and the dorsal prominence of the triquetrum is the location of the triangular fibrocartilage complex (TFCC; Figure 4-18). The central disk component supports the carpus, whereas the fibrous ligaments stabilize the DRUJ. Tenderness at the TFCC implies a degenerative or traumatic tear. Degenerative changes commonly occur with age and in individuals who have an ulnar length that exceeds the radial length, known as *ulnar-positive variance*. Acute tears can occur following

a fall. Tenderness can also be tested on the volar aspect of the TFCC, just proximal to the pisiform and under the flexor carpi ulnaris (FCU) tendon. In this region, the volar ulnocarpal ligaments contribute to the TFCC structure. Finally, TFCC tenderness can be noted directly on the ulnar aspect of the wrist beyond the head of the ulna and between the FCU and extensor carpi ulnaris (ECU) tendons. This region, sometimes referred to as the *mini snuffbox*, also contains the ulnar styloid, which can become tender following fracture or nonunion. Stability of the DRUJ, as determined primarily by the integrity of the TFCC, is best tested by stabilizing the distal radius and carpus with one hand, on the radial aspect of the wrist, and translating the neck of the ulna in the volar and dorsal direction with the other hand. Pain and relative motion between the ulnar head and the radius should be assessed and compared to the other side, because the joint normally subluxes a few millimeters. The joint should be completely stable with the wrist in full pronation and full supination. The test can also be performed by looking for the "piano key" volar or dorsal shift of the head of the ulna as the patient pushes the hand down on a table with an outstretched arm or pushes the hand up against resistance.

## PROVOCATIVE CARPAL TESTING FOR INSTABILITY AND ARTHRITIS

Normal function of the wrist depends on pain-free motion and stability. Trauma and inflammatory conditions can disrupt the intrinsic ligaments of the wrist, resulting in instability and eventual degenerative changes (De Smet, 2002). Similarly, trauma and inflammation that directly affect the cartilage surfaces of the carpus can also result in degeneration. The proximal carpal row—consisting of the scaphoid, lunate, and triquetrum—function as a unit that allows radiocarpal articulation but also provides a concavity to support and allow motion of the distal carpal row. For the proximal row to work as a unit, the scapholunate and lunotriquetral ligaments must be intact.

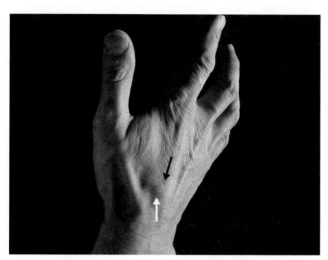

**FIGURE 4-16   THE BASE OF THE SECOND METACARPAL.** This is felt as a prominence (black arrow). It becomes increased in size with age and arthritis. The second CMC joint and trapezoid bone are proximal to the metacarpal base (white arrow).

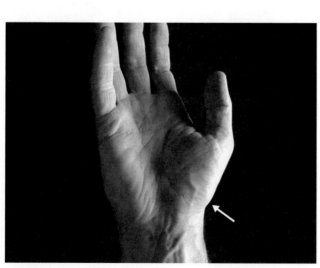

**FIGURE 4-17   FIRST CMC JOINT.** The joint is best palpated by using the pulps of the thumb in index finger, while the metacarpal is put through a range of motion with axial loading and attempted subluxation.

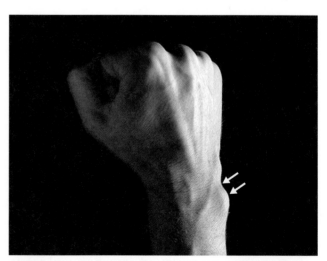

**FIGURE 4-18   THE TRIANGULAR FIBROCARTILAGE COMPLEX.** The TFCC is palpated with the tip or side of the examiner's finger on the dorsum in the sulcus between the ulnar head and triquetrum (top arrow) distal to the ulnar head (bottom arrow). It can also be palpated proximal to the pisiform.

### Scapholunate Ligament

Flexion of the scaphoid with radial deviation of the hand is a normal motion of the proximal row that cannot be overcome by the examiner's finger in the scaphoid tubercle (Beckenbaugh, 1984) (Figure 4-19). If it can be overcome, or if the scaphoid is ballotable, scapholunate ligament (SLL) laxity or tears are probable. The Watson test is performed by applying pressure on the flexed scaphoid tubercle while moving the hand back into ulnar deviation. Sudden and sharp dorsal wrist pain during this test indicates a significant SLL tear, resulting in instability and eventual osteoarthritis.

### Midcarpal Instability

This instability is characterized by vague, fatigue-like aching pain or a painful clunk with certain positions and is tested by stabilizing the radius with one hand and volarly translocating the carpus by pushing down on the hamate or capitate on the dorsum of the wrist (Figure 4-20). The wrist is reduced by bringing it into ulnar deviation, resulting in the "catch-up clunk" (Lichtman, 1984). Subluxation of the wrist is present in virtually everyone, but tenderness, pain, or reproduction of symptoms is important in the diagnosis of this type of instability.

## TENDONS AT THE WRIST

The 24 tendons around the wrist are examined by their predictable location. Tendon inflammation occurs in certain age groups and with excessive use. Crepitus and swelling are noted with acute inflammation but are less common with the chronic pain that can plague the tendons. All tendons are tested while assessing for pain by stretching the tendon, palpating it, and testing it against resistance.

The first of six dorsal extensor compartments is at the radial styloid region of the wrist and contains the abductor pollicis longus and extensor pollicis brevis tendons. Inflammation here, known as **de Quervain tenosynovitis,** is assessed with the **Finkelstein test** (Finkelstein, 1930 and Field, 1979), in which the thumb is held in the palm by the patient's flexed fingers as the wrist is passively brought into ulnar deviation. The maneuver reproduces the pain over the distal radius and the radial side of the wrist.

Inflammation of the extensor carpi radialis longus (ECRL) and brevis (ECRB) can occur in individuals who perform repetitive extension of the wrist, such as rowers. Pain is located at the junction where the two tendons emerge from under the muscles of the first compartment, approximately 3 cm proximal to the Lister tubercle on the dorsum of the distal radius (Wood, 1973). Inflammation here is known as **intersection syndrome.** The ECRL, and less commonly the ECRB, can also become inflamed at their insertion sites at the bases of the second and third metacarpals, respectively.

The extensor pollicis longus of the third compartment becomes inflamed at the Lister tubercle following minimally displaced distal radius fractures. In such cases, the tendon can quickly rupture, leading to a loss of extension of the IP joint of the thumb. The region can also become inflamed *de novo*, a condition known as **Drummer boy's palsy.**

Inflammation of the extensor digitorum communis and extensor indicis proprius of the fourth compartment occurs most commonly with inflammatory arthritis. This is a frequent finding in rheumatoid arthritis (RA). Inflammation of the extensor digiti minimi of the fifth compartment is rare but can occur with arthritis from the DRUJ, which is directly beneath the compartment. In RA, **rupture of the extensor tendons** for the fingers at the wrist results in loss of active extension at the MCP joint (finger drop).

The sixth compartment contains the extensor carpi ulnaris. The most common malady affecting this tendon is **subluxation,** tested by manually attempting to sublux the tendon out of its groove between the ulnar head and ulnar styloid.

Both of the two wrist flexors can become symptomatic with repetitive or excessive flexion. The flexor carpi radialis (FCR) typically becomes inflamed on the ulnar side of the scaphoid tubercle, where it travels down and into a tunnel at

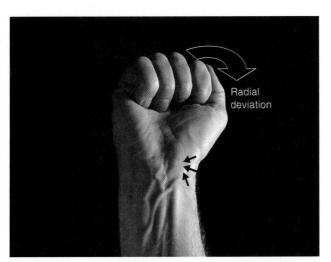

**FIGURE 4-19** The scaphoid tubercle becomes more prominent (black arrows) as the scaphoid flexes and the wrist moves into radial deviation; the examiner can overcome this flexion only in cases of scapholunate ligament tear or laxity. A click and pain while returning to ulnar deviation is a positive Watson test and correlates to a scapholunate ligament tear.

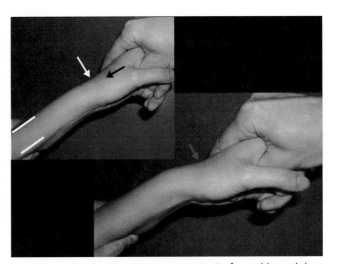

**FIGURE 4-20   THE MIDCARPAL CLUNK TEST.** Performed by stabilizing the radius (white bars) and translocating the wrist volarly (white arrow) while applying axial load (black arrow). Most wrists will sublux through the midcarpal joint with this maneuver (red arrow); a positive test is subluxation with reproduction of the patient's pain.

the trapezial ridge. The flexor carpi ulnaris (FCU) typically becomes inflamed proximal to the pisiform.

Inflammation of the nine flexor tendons of the digits (FDS, FDP, and FPL) usually occurs proximal to the wrist creases on the anterior aspect of the distal forearm. It is usually boggy in nature and is worse with finger motion.

## NERVES AT THE WRIST

The three major nerves at the wrist are assessed by percussion and compression and by assessing the appearance and power of the muscles that they innervate. The median nerve is percussed proximal to the flexor retinaculum, just radial to the palmaris longus tendon at the distal wrist crease. With symptomatic compression of the nerve in carpal tunnel syndrome, percussion produces paresthesia in the distribution of the nerve (**Tinel sign**) in the thumb, index, and middle fingers and the radial half of the ring finger. Sustained flexion of the wrist for 60 seconds can also induce finger paresthesias (**Phalen wrist flexion sign**). If the wrist cannot be flexed because of arthritis, pressure over the median nerve for 60 seconds often produces the same effect. The median nerve function is also assessed by gauging muscle atrophy and power of the thenar eminence (Palumbo, 2002).

**Ulnar nerve entrapment at the Guyon canal** can be assessed by compressing the ulnar nerve just radial to the pisiform for 1 minute. This produces numbness and tingling in the distribution of the ulnar nerve (positive ulnar nerve compression test). The Tinel sign will also be positive in the same distribution with percussion of the nerve. Prior to the wrist crease, the ulnar nerve gives off a sensory branch to the dorsal aspect of the hand. As such, sensory changes on the dorsum of the hand indicate more proximal compression of the nerve. Wasting may be noted in the intrinsic musculature of the hand as well as in the hypothenar eminence, depending on the site of compression. This may result in slight "clawing" of the little and ring fingers (hyperextension of MCP and flexion of PIP and DIP joints).

The superficial sensory branch of the radial nerve emerges from under the brachioradialis to innervate the dorsum of the radial two-thirds of the hand. **Wartenberg neuritis** of the nerve is assessed by percussion of the nerve in the region of the first compartment and radial styloid region. Neuritis can result from direct pressure or trauma, including a tight cast or splint, tight jewelry, or handcuffs.

## ARTERIES AT THE WRIST

In vascular disorders of the hand, the patency of the radial and ulnar arteries can be assessed using the Allen test: The patient elevates the hand and makes a fist while the examiner occludes both the radial and the ulnar arteries at the wrist. The patient then extends the fingers and repeats the maneuver until blanching of the hand is seen. Each artery is then released, and the color of the hand returns to normal. If either artery is occluded, the hand remains blanched when this artery alone is released. A marked difference between the left and right hand, or sluggish refill longer than 20 seconds, may indicate artery inflammation (**Buerger disease**) or traumatic thrombosis of the ulnar artery (**hypothenar hammer syndrome**).

# Injections of the Hand and Wrist

## INTRODUCTION

It is important to be aware of possible complications from steroid injections into tendons or joints. The risk of septic arthritis from intraarticular aspiration or injection is small, but common sense and aseptic technique must be adhered to within reason. The physician should wear gloves for his or her own protection, as body fluids from the patient can carry viral disease through small fissures or cuts into the caregiver. Where there is concern about overlying skin infection, such as cellulitis or septic bursitis, it is best to defer putting a needle into the joint.

With respect to the hand and wrist, some joints are very small, and a large volume of fluid injected into the articular cavity can stretch the capsule, even to the point of capsular herniation or rupture. Some joints (IP, wrist) and tendon sheaths are very difficult to aspirate, and the procedure is better done under ultrasound.

Repeated cortisone injections into the same site with great frequency may contribute to thinning of the articular cartilage, articular laxity, or tendon rupture due to protein catabolism, although reports of such complications are only anecdotal. Although very safe, it is important to understand that cortisone injections should not be the mainstay of management for ongoing disease. They can alleviate acute pain and inflammation, but when problems are ongoing, chronic, or frequently recurrent, other management strategies should be considered.

Finally, the patient should be forewarned that when an injection is placed close to the skin, such as at the wrist or PIP joint, the overlying skin may become atrophic or hypopigmented for many months, even as long as a year.

With the hand and wrist, after an articular injection is complete, the patient should be advised to keep the area clean and dry for 24 hours to avoid infection. Pain after injection occurs most often with tissue infiltration, such as for de Quervain syndrome. Along with analgesic tablets, ice in a plastic bag, applied on and off every 30 seconds, can provide relief. Where local anesthetic is infiltrated near a nerve (e.g., carpal tunnel syndrome), patients should be apprised of the possibility of paresthesia for a couple of hours afterward (Fam, 1995).

### Interphalangeal Joints

These joints are injected using a 25 gauge, 5/8 inch needle and a 1 mL syringe. Draw up 0.1 mL of local steroid and 0.1 mL of local anesthetic. The volume of injection should not exceed 0.3 mL to avoid stretching and damage of the capsule. Cadaveric studies have indicated that without ultrasound guidance, the needle is intraarticular in only 56% of cases; so if aspiration is important for diagnosis, ultrasound should be used (Raza et al, 2003). With the patient recumbent, the hand is placed palm down, fingers extended, on the examining table. For steroid injection the needle should be placed into the dorsomedial or dorsolateral aspect of the joint until the tip touches the articular cartilage. A slow injection is associated with slight ballooning of the capsule (Figure 4-21).

### Metacarpophalangeal Joints

MCP joints are injected using a 25 gauge, 5/8 inch needle and 1 mL syringe. Draw up 0.2 mL of local steroid and 0.1 mL of local anesthetic. The volume of the injection should not

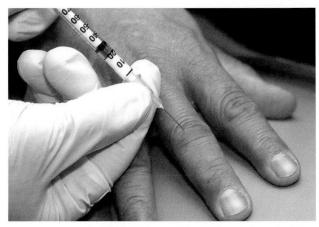

**FIGURE 4-21 INJECTION INTO PROXIMAL INTERPHALANGEAL JOINT OF THE FINGER.** The needle is placed just radial or ulnar to the extensor tendon and inserted into the joint margin.

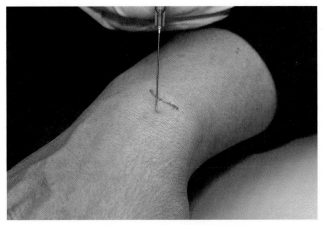

**FIGURE 4-23 INJECTION INTO WRIST USING LISTER TUBERCLE AS A LANDMARK (BLACK LINE).** Injection is placed 1 cm distal to this into the soft spot of the radioscaphoid joint.

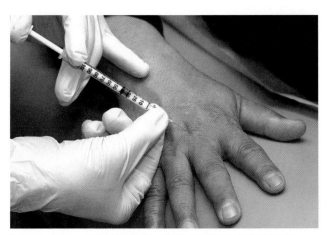

**FIGURE 4-22 INJECTION INTO METACARPOPHALANGEAL (MCP) JOINT.** Similar to PIP injection, the needle is inserted beside the extensor tendon as far as the joint margin.

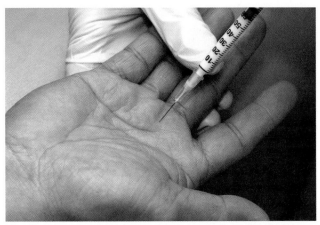

**FIGURE 4-24 INJECTION INTO FLEXOR TENDON OF FINGER.** Note: the injection can also be given starting in the palm, just proximal to the distal palmar crease, and aiming distally toward the finger.

exceed 0.4 mL to avoid stretching and damage of the capsule. The needle should be placed into the dorsomedial or dorsolateral aspect of the extended joint. As with the interphalangeal joint, it is often difficult to enter the intraarticular joint space. As the joint is injected, inflation of the capsule is palpable (Figure 4-22).

### Wrist Joint

The radiocarpal joint is best approached from the dorsum of the wrist. The patient is supine with the hand prone on the examining table. A 22 gauge, 1 or 1½ inch needle is used. Local anesthetic can be infiltrated as the needle is inserted. The landmark is the Lister tubercle at the distal end of the radius. About 1 cm distal to the turbercle is a soft spot that represents the space between the distal radius and the base of the scaphoid. The needle is inserted vertical to the wrist to a depth of 2 cm. If resistance is met, pull back halfway and direct a bit in a distal and radial direction. With the needle in place, the syringe is exchanged (sometimes a needle clamp is needed) for one with local steroid to a volume of 1 mL (Figure 4-23).

### Flexor Tendon (Saldana, 2001)

The patient is positioned recumbent, lying on the side to be injected, with the arm extended on the examining table and the hand held in a flat supine position. A 25 gauge, 5/8 inch needle can be used with a 1 mL syringe. The volume for injection should be about 0.6 mL. It may be helpful to mix 0.2 mL of local anesthetic with 0.4 mL of the injectable steroid.

The tendon to be injected is grasped between the thumb and forefinger of the examiner's free hand, about 1 cm proximal to the distal palmar crease. The needle is inserted vertical to the palm, aimed in a slightly distal direction. Initially the needle tip may be in the substance of the tendon, so resistance may be encountered. The examiner should withdraw the needle until the steroid flows smoothly and easily. The tendon sheath will balloon in a tubular fashion as the steroid is injected (Figure 4-24).

### de Quervain Syndrome

The first of six dorsal extensor compartments is at the radial styloid region of the wrist and contains the abductor pollicis longus and extensor pollicis brevis tendons. These tendons

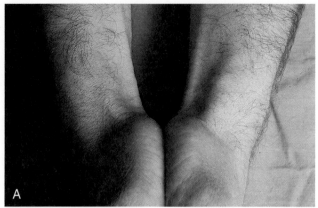

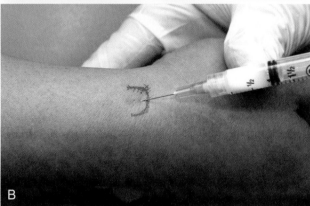

**FIGURE 4-25**  **A, de QUERVAIN TENOSYNOVITIS OF THE WRISTS.** (From Hochberg H, Silman AJ, Smolen JS, et al., eds.: *Rheumatology,* 3rd ed. London: Mosby, 2003.) **B, INJECTION INTO FIRST COMPARTMENT SHEATH FOR ABDUCTOR POLLICIS LONGUS AND EXTENSOR POLLICIS BREVIS.** Line marks margin of radial styloid.

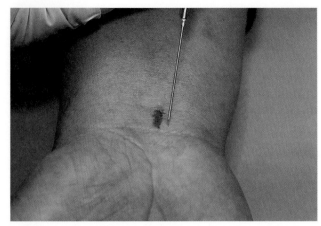

**FIGURE 4-26**  **INJECTION INTO CARPAL TUNNEL.** Note needle placement on ulnar side of palmaris longus as marked (black line).

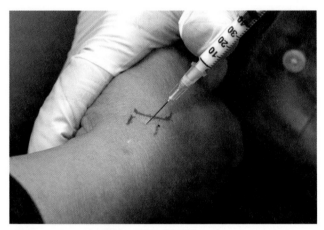

**FIGURE 4-27**  **INJECTION INTO CARPOMETACARPAL JOINT OF THUMB.** Lines mark base of proximal phalanx, abductor pollicis longus, and extensor carpi radialis tendons.

are held in place by a vaginal sheath. Inflammation here is known as **de Quervain syndrome** (Figure 4-25A). Injection is placed into the sheath with a 25 gauge, 5/8 inch needle. A 3 mL Luer lock syringe is filled with 0.5 mL of local steroid and 0.5 mL of local anesthetic. With the wrist in ulnar deviation, the needle is inserted on the radial aspect of the wrist at the radial styloid, about 3 cm proximal to the base of the first metacarpal. The needle is inserted in a slightly proximal direction, aiming toward the elbow, until resistance is met; the needle tip is pulled back slightly until the solution can be injected with little resistance. The sheath should swell slightly with the injection (see Figure 4-25B).

### Carpal Tunnel Syndrome

Injection into the carpal tunnel may relieve compression of the median nerve only temporarily. The palmaris longus tendon insertion is identified at the proximal palmar crease with resisted flexion of the third finger. A 22 gauge, 1 to 1½ inch needle is used with a 3 mL syringe. One mL of local steroid and a half mL of local anesthetic can be used. The needle is inserted just ulnar to the palmaris longus, at the proximal palmar crease, at a 20° to 30° angle to the skin, aimed toward the fourth finger (Figure 4-26). Snagging on a flexor tendon can occur, at which point the needle should be withdrawn slightly and reangled. The needle should be inserted to 2 cm. The anesthetic may leave some

tingling in the median nerve distribution for a couple of hours.

### First Carpometacarpal Joint

The base of the first metacarpal is identified at the distal end of the anatomical snuffbox between the abductor pollicis longus and the extensor pollicis brevis (EPB) tendons. Flexion of the thumb across the palm makes the joint easier to identify. A 1 mL syringe with a 25 gauge, 5/8 inch needle can be used. About 0.3 mL of local steroid should be mixed with 0.1 mL of local anesthetic. The needle is inserted perpendicular to the skin close to the EPB tendon to avoid the radial artery. Traction on the thumb can sometimes open up the joint space for better access (Figure 4-27).

### Distal Radioulnar Joint

The groove between the distal radius and distal ulna can be identified with palpation while passively supinating and pronating the hand. The injection is placed about 1 cm proximal to the groove, where the joint has a synovial pouch. A 3 mL syringe with a 22 gauge, 1 or 1½ inch needle should be used. A half mL of local anesthetic should be mixed with 1 mL of local steroid. The injection needle is inserted perpendicular to the wrist to a depth of about 2.5 cm.

# REFERENCES

Beckenbaugh, R.D., 1984. Accurate evaluation and management of the painful wrist following injury. An approach to carpal instability. Orthop. Clin. North Am. 15, 289–306.

De Smet, L., 2002. Classification for congenital anomalies of the hand: the IFSSH classification and the JSSH modification. Genetic Counseling 13 (3), 331–8.

Fam, A.G., 1995. Aspiration and injection of joints and periarticular tissues: The wrist and hand. In: Klippel, J.H., Dieppe, P.A. (Eds.), Practical Rheumatology, first ed. Mosby, London, pp. 117–118.

Fam, A.G., 2003. The wrist and hand. In: Hochberg, H., Silman, A.J., Smolen, J.S. (Eds.), Rheumatology, third ed. Mosby, London, pp. 641–650.

Field, J.H., 1979. de Quervain's disease. Am. Fam. Physician 20, 103–104.

Finkelstein, H., 1930. Stenosing tendovaginitis at the radial styloid process. J. Bone Joint Surg. (Am) 12, 509–540.

Lichtman, D.M., Noble III, W.H., Alexander, C.E., 1984. Dynamic triquetrolunate instability: case report. J. Hand Surg. (Am) 9, 185–188.

Markison, R.E., Kilgore, E.S., 1987. Hand. In: Davis, J.H. (Ed.), Clinical Surgery, CV Mosby, St. Louis, pp. 2292–2353.

McMurtry, R.Y., 1986. The hand. In: Little, A.H. The Rheumatological Physical Examination. Grune & Stratton, Orlando, FL, pp. 91–100.

Palumbo, C.F., Szabo, R.M., 2002. Examination of patients for carpal tunnel syndrome: Sensibility, provocative, and motor testing. Hand Clin. 18, 269–277.

Raza, K., Lee, C.Y., Pilling, D., et al., 2003. Ultrasound guidance allows accurate needle placement and aspiration from small joints in patients with early inflammatory arthritis. Rheumatology 42, 976–979.

Saar, J.D., Grothaus, P.C., 2000. Dupuytren's disease: An overview. Plast. Reconstruct. Surg. 106, 125–134.

Saldana, M.J., 2001. Trigger digits: Diagnosis and treatment. J. Am. Acad. Orthop. Surg. 9, 246–252.

Strauch, B., de Moura, W., 1985. Digital flexor tendon sheath: An anatomic study. J. Hand Surg. Am. 10, 785–810.

von Schroeder, H.P., Botte, M.J., 1993. The functional significance of the long extensors and juncturae tendinum in finger extension. J. Hand Surg. [Am] 18 (4), 641–647.

von Schroeder, H.P., Botte, M.J., 1997. Functional anatomy of the extensor tendons of the digits. Hand Clin. 13 (1), 51–62.

Watson, H.K., Ashmead, D.I.V., Makhouf, M.V., 1988. Examination of the scaphoid. J. Hand Surg. (Am) 13 (5), 657–660.

Wood, M.B., Linscheid, R.L., 1973. Abductor pollicis longus bursitis. Clin. Orthop. 93, 293–296.

# 5

# THE HIP

Hans J. Kreder • Dana Jerome

## Applied Anatomy

The low back, sacroiliac joint, and hip joints can all cause pain in a similar anatomic distribution, and each must be considered in the evaluation of a patient with complaints of pain in the region of the lower back, buttock, groin, or knee. Pain from the hip joint is poorly localized and may be felt in the groin, inner thigh, trochanteric area, buttock, anterior thigh, and/or knee.

The morphology of the sacroiliac (SI) joint varies considerably with age, among individuals, and even from side to side in the same individual. It represents the largest paraxial joint, with a surface area of more than 17 cm$^2$ in adults. The anteroinferior ventral part of the SI joint is synovial, whereas the posterosuperior part is a fibrous joint supported by powerful ligaments. The joint is surrounded by a thin capsule that may be absent posteriorly. Little movement occurs at the SI joint (Figure 5-1; see also Figure 8-6 in Chapter 8). The SI joint is innervated by the L5 and S1 through S4 nerve roots.

### HIP JOINT

The hip joint is a ball-and-socket, weight-bearing articulation that combines a wide range of motion (ROM) with considerable stability. The stability of the joint depends on the deep insertion of the femoral head into the acetabular socket, the strong capsule and ligaments, the powerful muscles surrounding the joints, and the circular fibrocartilaginous **acetabular labrum.** The latter forms a tight ring around the femoral head. The **capsule** is attached proximally to the edge of the acetabulum, acetabular labrum, and transverse ligament, which bridges the acetabular notch inferiorly. Distally, the capsule is attached to the intertrochanteric line anteriorly and to the femoral neck about 1.5 cm proximal to the intertrochanteric crest posteriorly. It follows, therefore, that a large part of the femoral neck is intracapsular.

The anterior capsule is reinforced by the powerful Y-shaped **iliofemoral ligament,** which prevents excessive hip extension and external rotation (Figure 5-2). The weaker posterior capsule is reinforced by the thinner **ischiofemoral ligament,** which prevents excessive external rotation, and the **pubofemoral ligament,** which opposes excessive hip abduction (see Figure 5-2). The **ligamentum femoris teres**—which is a channel for blood vessels to the femoral head, is located between the pit of the femoral head and the transverse ligament of the acetabulum. It provides little stability but nourishes a small area of the femoral head adjacent to the

attachment of the ligament. Therefore, dislocation of the femoral head from the acetabulum is resisted primarily by the acetabular labrum and by the strong hip joint capsule, which incorporates the capsular Y ligament (see Figure 5-2). The fibers of the hip joint capsule are wound around the femoral neck so as to tighten with hip extension and internal rotation (Figure 5-3). The position is uncomfortable for patients with hip arthritis because of tension on the capsular structures. The intracapsular space of the hip joint is smallest with the hip in extension and internal rotation, a position that produces maximum tension on the capsular Y ligament. Consequently, patients with inflammation of the hip joint often hold the extremity flexed and externally rotated as a position of relative comfort.

The **iliotibial band** is a thickened band in the fascia lata that connects the iliac crest to the **Gerdy tubercle.** It is attached to the entire length of the intermuscular septum between the vastus lateralis and the hamstring muscles over the greater trochanter. It is a mechanical tie between the iliac crest, sacrum, and ischial tuberosity proximally and between the lateral femoral and tibial condyles, particularly to the Gerdy tubercle on the anterolateral aspect of the proximal tibia, and the head of the fibula distally.

The **synovial membrane** lines the inner surface of the capsule and covers the acetabular labrum, ligamentum femoris teres, and parts of the femoral neck. There are three main bursae around the hip joint. The **trochanteric bursa** is the largest. It is a multiloculated bursa between the gluteus maximus and the greater trochanter. The **ischiogluteal bursa** lies between the gluteus maximus and ischial tuberosity. The gluteus maximus covers the ischial tuberosity in the neutral position, but with hip flexion, both the tuberosity and the bursa become uncovered. The **iliopectineal bursa** lies in the middle third of the inguinal region, between the iliofemoral and pubofemoral ligaments; in relation to the iliopsoas muscle and tendon, it lies just lateral to the femoral artery. The bursa communicates with the hip joint in about 15% of adults, and in patients with hip arthritis, it can manifest as a fluid-distended, cystic swelling in the groin.

Having the femoral head situated in an offset position on the femoral shaft, through the femoral neck, minimizes bony impingement and maximizes normal hip ROM. It does, however, require strong muscular support to stabilize the trunk over the hip joints, especially in single-leg stance phase, when the body's center of gravity is medial to the supporting leg. One can consider the hip joint as a fulcrum for a lever, with the body's center of gravity acting

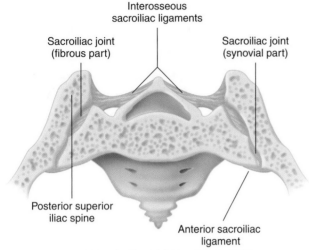

Interosseous
sacroiliac ligaments

Sacroiliac joint
(fibrous part)

Sacroiliac joint
(synovial part)

Posterior superior
iliac spine

Anterior sacroiliac
ligament

**FIGURE 5-1   CROSS-SECTION OF THE PELVIS SHOWING THE ANATOMY OF THE SACROILIAC JOINT.**

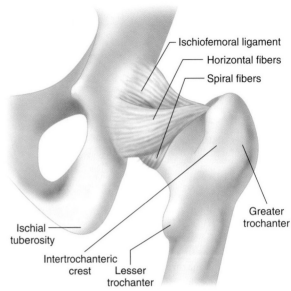

Ischiofemoral ligament

Horizontal fibers

Spiral fibers

Greater
trochanter

Ischial
tuberosity

Intertrochanteric
crest

Lesser
trochanter

**FIGURE 5-3   CAPSULAR STRUCTURES OF THE HIP JOINT: POSTERIOR ASPECT.**

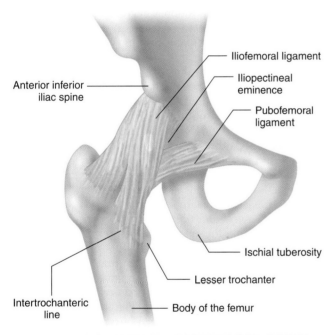

Iliofemoral ligament

Iliopectineal
eminence

Pubofemoral
ligament

Anterior inferior
iliac spine

Ischial tuberosity

Lesser trochanter

Intertrochanteric
line

Body of the femur

**FIGURE 5-2   CAPSULAR STRUCTURES OF THE HIP JOINT: ANTERIOR ASPECT.**

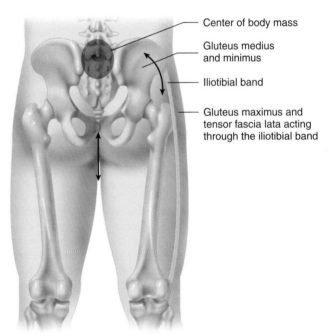

Center of body mass

Gluteus medius
and minimus

Iliotibial band

Gluteus maximus and
tensor fascia lata acting
through the iliotibial band

**FIGURE 5-4   HIP BIOMECHANICS DURING SINGLE-LEG STANCE.**
(From Gross J, Fetto J, Rosen E., eds.: *Musculoskeletal Examination*, 2nd ed. Malden, MA: Blackwell Publishing, 2002.)

approximately 1 cm anterior to the first sacral segment in the midline (Figure 5-4). To counteract this load, the gluteus medius and minimus act in conjunction with the tensor fascia lata and gluteus maximus muscles, which function mainly through their insertion into the iliotibial band. Given the fact that the distance is twice as far to the center of gravity as it is to the gluteus insertion into the proximal femur, a force approximately equal to three times body weight is transmitted through the hip joint during single-leg stance, compared with one half of the body weight during normal bilateral stance (Figure 5-5).

On anteroposterior radiographs of the hip, the normal femoral neck–shaft angle in an adult is 120° to 135°. In coxa vara the angle is less than 120°; in coxa valga, the angle is greater than 135°.

## Hip Pain and History Taking

Patients who complain of hip pain often mean very different things, from pain in the lower back or buttock region to groin pain or thigh pain. Patients with true hip joint disease will classically complain of pain in the groin region, although this varies depending on the type of hip pathology. Pain typically radiates down toward the anterior aspect of the knee. Individuals who are experiencing pain on the lateral aspect of the hip, in the region of the greater trochanter, or pain in the lower back or in the buttock area may

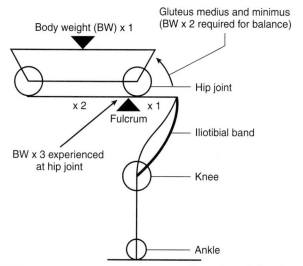

**FIGURE 5-5    HIP BIOMECHANICS: FORCES.** (From Gross J, Fetto J, Rosen E., eds.: *Musculoskeletal Examination*, 2nd ed. Malden, MA: Blackwell Publishing, 2002.)

also complain of hip pain. To determine what the patient's complaint of "hip pain" really means, it is essential to ask the patient to describe exactly where the pain is primarily located and where it radiates. Other than pain, the patient may complain of limited function, stiffness, limping, and audible or palpable clicking or snapping noises about the hip. As with any history, it is important to delineate the onset of these symptoms, their severity, whether they were preceded by injury or overuse, and whether there are any constitutional or systemic symptoms. Inflammatory arthritis generally affects multiple joints, and although the hip may be the presenting problem, it is important to inquire about similar symptoms in any other joints. It is essential to inquire about childhood hip problems, previous injuries, and the nature of any previous hip or spinal operations.

Symptoms in this region may originate from the hip or from the spine, SI joint, or soft tissues surrounding the hip, or it may be referred from a remote site. Occasionally a patient complains only of pain that is deep-seated about the knee joint, and the underlying hip pathology may be missed if the examination concentrates solely on the knee. As part of the physical examination, it is essential to evaluate other regions that may be the source of referred pain. Typically, the joint above and below an area that a patient is complaining about should be examined. For the hip joint this requires that the lower back and sacroiliac region, as well as the knee joint, be evaluated.

It is also useful to assess the magnitude of functional impairment and disability and the severity of the pain. This can be done using validated pain scales and functional measurement instruments, such as the Western Ontario and McMaster Universities (WOMAC) Osteoarthritis Index. A clear understanding of the patient's occupational, sports, recreational, and social activities and how the hip problem affects the patient's quality of life is essential to the consideration of how a potential treatment might be planned so as to optimize patient function in light of the individual's unique needs.

Based on the patient's history, the clinician will generally have some idea what is generating the patient's hip pain. A full hip examination should be performed along with examination of the knee and the back. A good history can guide the clinician toward the appropriate special tests on physical examination that will help accurately diagnose the patient's problem. For example, if the patient tells you that the focus of their pain is in the lateral aspect of the hip, it will be important to palpate the greater trochanter for tenderness, looking for signs of trochanteric bursitis.

## Common Painful Disorders of the Hip Region

### OSTEOARTHRITIS AND INFLAMMATORY HIP ARTHRITIS

Hip arthritis typically causes pain in the groin or low buttock area, with possible radiation into the knee. The pain in osteoarthritis is generally worse with activity and is relieved by rest. In inflammatory arthritis, the patient may experience stiffness with inactivity and some improvement of this symptom with movement of the hip joint. Some patients experience very little pain but complain of stiffness, limping, and functional decline. The onset of pain and functional decline can be quite insidious, occurring over many years. Some patients consider these progressive symptoms to represent part of normal aging and do not seek help until quite late in the disease process. Functionally, the combination of stiffness and pain leads to complaints of a limp, difficulty getting up out of low chairs, difficulty descending and ascending stairs (requiring 36° and 67° of flexion respectively), inability to squat (120° of flexion, 20° of abduction, and 20° of hip external rotation required), and trouble with daily activities, such as putting on socks and shoes.

Physical findings may include a combined Trendelenburg and antalgic gait, actual or functional shortening of the limb due to collapse of the hip joint, and soft-tissue contractures around the hip joint. Early hip joint arthritis is associated with pain on hip extension and internal rotation, as the capsule tightens, and early loss of internal rotation in flexion and extension. Fixed flexion deformity and limited abduction and adduction are common with more advanced disease.

### TROCHANTERIC BURSITIS

This condition is extremely common. The greater trochanteric bursa may become inflamed due to direct trauma or overuse with strenuous physical activity, such as running or jumping. A tight iliotibial tract, with a positive Ober test, may be present. The inflamed bursa becomes painful with activities that compress it between the greater trochanter and the overlying iliotibial band. Patients may be unable to lie on the affected side, and they usually experience pain with weight bearing, especially in a single-leg stance, as the iliotibial band tightens to maintain the body's upright posture. Tenderness over the greater trochanter with direct palpation and pain with resisted hip abduction are typical physical findings. A fluid-distended bursa associated with a palpable fluctuant swelling may be palpated on rare occasions in a thin patient.

## SNAPPING HIP (COXA SALTANS)

Young patients may present with complaints of snapping or clicking about the hip. Some may believe that the hip is dislocating, which is highly unlikely without significant trauma or underlying hip joint arthroplasty. Snapping or clicking about the hip can be caused by intraarticular pathology or by causes external to the hip joint. **Intraarticular causes** include loose bodies (synovial chondromatosis, fracture fragments, broken-off osteophytes), labrum tears, and, rarely, a true subluxing hip joint, especially after total hip replacement surgery. Intraarticular clicking caused by loose bodies may be intermittent and can sometimes be demonstrated during active and passive ROM testing. If a labrum tear is suspected, internal rotation of the flexed hip in adduction with axial compression may cause pain. **Extraarticular causes** are far more common; they include sliding of the iliotibial band or fibers of the gluteus maximus muscle over the greater trochanter and, less commonly, snapping of the iliopsoas tendon over the femoral head. Generalized ligamentous laxity is a common finding in these individuals. The patient can often demonstrate the clicking voluntarily by active movement of the hip, and the underlying snapping or clicking can often be felt laterally over the greater trochanter, as the iliotibial band snaps back and forth. Palpable, and sometimes audible, medial clicking from the iliopsoas tendon is best demonstrated during active hip flexion and external rotation, followed by active hip extension.

## PERIARTICULAR FRACTURE

A displaced hip fracture through the subcapital or intertrochanteric region is a dramatic event that results in sudden severe pain and inability to bear weight or to move the affected hip. Most acetabular or pelvic fractures are the result of high-energy trauma with an equally dramatic presentation that allows ready diagnosis of the problem.

A fall in an elderly patient can lead to complaints of hip pain that may be due simply to soft-tissue injury, stable lateral compression pelvic fracture, undisplaced subcapital hip fracture, or a fracture of the acetabular dome region. These fractures, especially acetabular dome fractures, are easily missed, even on plain radiographs. Careful physical examination and a high index of suspicion should lead to appropriate investigations, such as a CT scan, that can help to confirm the diagnosis. Usually the history involves a low-energy traumatic event, but in the case of a fragility fracture through osteoporotic bone, there may be no history of trauma whatsoever. The patient may have difficulty bearing weight on the affected extremity, but in some cases, patients have been known to walk on a fractured hip for many weeks before the diagnosis is made.

Physical examination may reveal bruising and tenderness over the greater trochanter, suggesting local trauma. With **undisplaced or minimally displaced subcapital hip fractures,** the findings may be quite subtle: limb shortening; external rotation deformity; pain on internal rotation, which tightens the capsule; global reduction in ROM due to pain; and, often, difficulty initiating a straight leg lift (inability to lift the heel of the extended lower extremity off the examining table because of the forces generated across the hip joint during this activity). Striking the heel of the extended leg with the examiner's fist is usually quite painful in the presence of a subcapital or acetabular dome fracture, but this maneuver typically does not cause pain with soft-tissue bruising, because the involved soft tissues are not moved or stretched. To look for possible subcapital femoral neck fractures, the proximal femur should be imaged in the anteroposterior plane with the hip in internal rotation to better visualize the entire length of the femoral neck (considering that the femoral neck is anteverted relative to the femoral shaft). A lateral radiograph of the proximal femur should also be obtained and assessed for fracture angulation. **Stable compression pelvic fractures** can be diagnosed by tenderness to palpation anteriorly along the pubic ramus and posteriorly along the sacrum and SI region. Compressing the pelvis by pushing the two iliac crests together usually increases pelvic pain.

Plain radiographs of the pelvis, including inlet and outlet views, are required to confirm the examiner's suspicion of a lateral compression pelvic fracture. If plain radiographs do not show evidence of proximal femoral or pelvic fracture, and suspicion for a significant bony injury remains, a CT scan of the acetabular dome and proximal femur should be obtained, because plain films usually do not reveal the presence of an acetabular dome fracture.

## SACROILIAC JOINT PAIN

Inflammation of the SI joint (sacroiliitis) can be the source of buttock and upper thigh pain. This is seen classically as ankylosing spondylitis and the other seronegative spondyloarthropathies. The combination of maximal pain below L5 plus pain in the region of the **posterior superior iliac spine** (PSIS) and tenderness in the sacral sulcus region has a positive predictive value of 60%. The classic feature of sacroiliitis on history is that the back pain is improved with activity and exacerbated by rest. This pain will usually waken a patient from sleep at night. SI imaging, plain films, or MRI can be used for definitive evaluation of the SI joint. On physical examination it will be important to stress the SI joint with a flexion abduction external rotation (FABER) test.

## OSTEITIS PUBIS

Pain in the region of the anterior pelvis due to inflammation and erosive lesions of the symphysis pubis, or **osteitis pubis,** is an uncommon disorder of diverse causes that include spondyloarthropathies, trauma, infection, distance running, and multiple deliveries. The condition is characterized by insidious-onset midline anterior pain that may radiate to either groin. The pain is exacerbated by passive abduction and resisted adduction of the hip, and tenderness is found on palpation over the anterior border of the symphysis pubis and adjacent pubic rami; exacerbation with pelvic internal and external stress is also seen.

## CONSIDERATIONS IN PATIENTS AFTER TOTAL HIP REPLACEMENT

### Safety Considerations

Special care should be taken when evaluating the hip joint of a patient who has previously undergone total hip replacement. In the early postoperative period, the clinician should ask patients whether their surgeon has informed them of any specific restrictions. For example, hip revision surgery may involve compromise to the hip abductor muscles, and active hip abduction may be contraindicated in the early postoperative period. Similarly, patients may be instructed to avoid weight bearing during the initial 6 weeks after complex revision hip reconstructive surgery and occasionally after uncemented or complicated primary hip replacement surgery. Hip precautions in the early postoperative period are meant to minimize the risk of hip dislocation, although with the newer surgical techniques, these restrictions are being relaxed. The restrictions involve limiting hip flexion beyond 90°, internal rotation of the hip in flexion, external rotation of the hip in extension, and hip adduction beyond the midline. When testing ROM, the risk of anterior dislocation of the hip is greatest with the hip in extension, adduction, and external rotation. The risk of posterior dislocation is greatest when the hip is flexed, internally rotated, and adducted.

### Leg Lengths

In the early postoperative period after total hip replacement surgery, the clinician should be careful with respect to the evaluation of leg lengths. Hip arthritis is commonly associated with joint collapse, fixed flexion deformity, and adductor tendon contraction that leads to significant functional shortening of the involved lower extremity. The limb may initially appear functionally long to the patient after surgery, given the correction of the deformity that is achieved intraoperatively. Residual soft-tissue contractures about the ipsilateral or contralateral hip, or pelvic tilt secondary to degenerative scoliosis, may also give the patient the perception of having a relatively short or long lower limb after surgery. Even if a small, true leg-length discrepancy is discovered after careful examination, it may be best to wait for at least 6 months after hip replacement surgery before recommending corrective shoe raises or inserts. This time frame allows for some contractures to resolve, and many patients will no longer require leg-length adjustment.

## Pain after Total Hip Arthroplasty

Although a comprehensive review of the evaluation of the painful total hip replacement is beyond the scope of this chapter, the following possible causes are considered.

### MECHANICAL FAILURE

Hip dislocation and periprosthetic femur or acetabular fracture typically result in severe functional impairment, usually with complete inability to walk, severe pain, and often characteristic deformity. The emergency management of these conditions is similar to that for a traumatic hip joint dislocation or femur fracture and includes a thorough neurovascular examination.

### INSTABILITY OF THE ARTICULATION

Complete dislocation can be associated with spontaneous reduction. The patient may recall sudden groin pain, sometimes associated with a "clunking" sound or sensation. **Anterior subluxation** commonly occurs when the ipsilateral leg is planted on the ground, and the upper body rotates to the opposite side, resulting in relative extension and external rotation, often also with adduction, of the ipsilateral hip. Typically, the anteriorly dislocated hip lies in an abducted and externally rotated position. **Posterior subluxation** is more common and can occur while the patient is lying in bed on the opposite side with the ipsilateral hip flexed, adducted, and externally rotated. Typically, the posteriorly dislocated hip lies in an adducted and internally rotated position. A "push-pull" test can be safely performed to assess the soft-tissue tension around an artificial hip joint. This involves stabilizing the pelvis and placing the hip in extension, neutral rotation, and abduction. The examiner attempts to distract the hip joint by applying a traction force to the limb and then pushing it back into place. Very little movement should be detectable through the hip joint.

### IMPLANT LOOSENING AND INFECTION

Loosening of the implant–bone interface may be associated with pain. Important causes of loosening include traumatic mechanisms, osteolysis due to implant wear, and infection. The examiner should inquire about recent falls or other injuries and the relationship of these events to the onset of pain. Information regarding how long the hip replacement has been in situ can provide clues regarding the possibility of implant wear. Finally, potential sources of infection and its systemic manifestations should be sought. Low-grade infections may go undetected for many months before implant loosening or systemic manifestations are noted. Typically, pain due to infection is always present and is not relieved with rest, whereas mechanical loosening may result in intermittent pain, usually with activity. Pain in the groin region is more commonly associated with acetabular implant problems, including loosening or impingement, and thigh pain is more commonly seen with loosening of the femoral component. When the patient is arising from a low chair, a considerable force is placed on the femoral component, which may rotate slightly when loose and cause pain.

### BURSITIS

Trochanteric bursitis is common after total hip replacement surgery, especially with lateral approaches that involve dissection of the soft tissues from the greater trochanter during surgery. Symptoms include pain with single-leg stance and with active hip abduction and discomfort when lying on the ipsilateral side. The trochanter is tender to palpation.

### TENDINITIS AND CONTRACTURES OF TENDONS AND MUSCLES

Before hip replacement surgery, contractures may have formed in the soft tissues around the hip as a consequence of arthritis-related joint stiffness. These muscles and tendons may become painful as a consequence of increased ROM and tension on the structures after successful joint replacement surgery that allows greater ROM. The hip abductors and flexors are most commonly affected. The patient may complain of a deep anteromedial or medial pain that is worse with active hip flexion or active adduction. Tenderness should be evaluated over specific tendons, although the iliopsoas tendon usually cannot be palpated because of its deep insertion. Pain with active contraction of the affected tendon–muscle unit and pain with passive stretch are consistent with the diagnosis of tendinitis.

## REFERRED AND UNRELATED PAIN

Patients with degenerative hip arthritis commonly also have lumbosacral spine arthritis. Persistent buttock and thigh pain may be referred from the lower spine or the SI joint. These patients may not manifest any signs of nerve root irritation. Other unrelated sources of pain may include groin hernias, peripheral vascular disease, meralgia paraesthetica, and metabolic disease such as Paget disease.

# Physical Examination

Patient evaluation is not a linear process but involves a constant reevaluation of clinical evidence gained from the history and physical assessment. It is impossible to record the specific order of evaluation that an experienced clinician might pursue, because it depends entirely on the unique presentation of the particular patient. By convention, the physical examination is presented as inspection, palpation, movement, and special tests. However, an experienced clinician moves fluidly back and forth through these evaluation modalities, gathering essential information and perhaps also asking additional questions as new evidence emerges. The clinician should have some knowledge as to the sensitivity and specificity of the clinical evaluation maneuvers being performed, so that the most useful tests are considered first. Another basic principle is to minimize patient change in position as much as possible, especially in a patient with significant discomfort or difficulty during movement. Therefore, while the patient is standing, all relevant examinations requiring this posture might be undertaken before the patient is asked to lie on the examining table. Then, all tests that require the supine position are done before the patient is asked to move to the lateral decubitus position and, finally, to the prone position.

## INSPECTION

The evaluation requires that the patient be undressed down to shorts or underwear, including removal of shoes and socks. One should consider having a family member or a health care professional of the same gender present during the examination, especially if the patient seems ill at ease.

Inspection always begins with an evaluation of the patient as a whole, or a **general inspection.** Are there clues as to the presence of a chronic systemic condition, such as rheumatoid arthritis? Is the patient generally fit in appearance, or is he or she above ideal body weight for height? **Localized inspection** involves an assessment of the following:

1. **Skin and superficial tissues:** Skin incisions or scars should be explained, and any relationship to the current symptoms should be explored. Skin discoloration, ulceration, and distal hair loss may be associated with vascular insufficiency. Characteristic psoriatic skin and nail lesions are helpful clues.

2. **Deep tissue:** Evaluation should include the subcutaneous tissues and muscles. Asymmetric swelling over one greater trochanter may be associated with underlying trochanteric bursitis. An abdominal pannus (apron) may cause meralgia paraesthetica, a condition in which the lateral femoral cutaneous nerve becomes compressed as it runs beneath the lateral end of the inguinal ligament, resulting in pain and numbness in the proximal lateral thigh. A cystic swelling in the middle third of the inguinal region may represent a fluid-distended, communicating iliopectineal bursa. Disuse atrophy of the proximal quadriceps muscle is common in hip arthritis. This can be assessed by tape measurement comparing the two sides. Asymmetry of the gluteus maximus or other muscles can be caused by peripheral nerve injury or nerve root impingement that causes muscle wasting.

3. **Bony landmarks:** The hip joint itself lies hidden from direct inspection, although assessment of surrounding bony landmarks can provide clues to the underlying hip pathology. These include the lumbosacral spinous processes, iliac crest, anterior superior iliac spine, greater trochanter, ischial tuberosity, posterior superior iliac spines, overlying "dimples of Venus," and symphysis pubis.

It is often easiest to divide the inspection portion of the exam into that which can be done with the patient standing and then that which should be done with the patient supine. With the patient standing, the examiner should inspect the patient's gait (see Gait Analysis). The examiner should then examine the standing patient from the front, from each side, and from the back. In this position it is easier to detect the presence of spinal curvature and pelvic tilts. These are assessed by examining the relationship between the adjacent spinous processes and the left and right iliac crests. A leg-length deformity may be apparent while the patient is standing with the feet together. If the patient needs to flex one knee to keep the pelvis level, the side with the flexed knee might be long. Conversely, if the pelvis is tilted to one side and the knees are fully extended, the side on which the pelvis is lower may be short. Gross varus or valgus deformity of the knee can also be evaluated (see Chapter 6). When the patient moves to a supine position, a more detailed inspection of skin, superficial, and deep tissues can be performed.

## GAIT ANALYSIS

Normal gait involves a complex integration of muscle and joint activity that results in forward propulsion of the body with minimum displacement in the vertical and horizontal planes. Each leg alternates between a **stance phase** and a **swing phase** (Figure 5-6). During normal gait, the stance phase accounts for approximately 60% of the gait cycle. With faster walking speed, stance time is reduced and swing time is increased. The stance phase includes heel strike, foot flat, midstance, heel lift, and toe lift. Swing phase begins after toe lift and involves an initial period of acceleration, followed by midswing and a period of deceleration before heel contact and the stance phase begin again.

Vertical displacement of the body's center of gravity is minimized by the following mechanisms: 1) a slight pelvic drop during midswing, after an initial rise of the pelvis on the unsupported side after toe lift; 2) pelvic rotation forward on the swing side; 3) ankle plantar flexion shortly after heel strike;

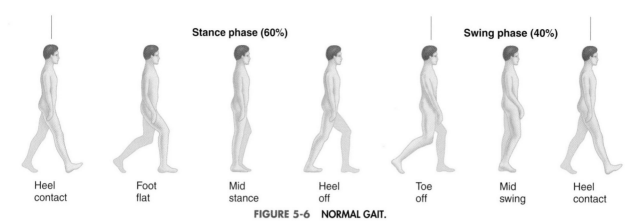

**Stance phase (60%)**          **Swing phase (40%)**

| Heel contact | Foot flat | Mid stance | Heel off | Toe off | Mid swing | Heel contact |

**FIGURE 5-6    NORMAL GAIT.**

4) stance phase knee flexion; and 5) ankle plantar flexion in preparation for toe lift. The body's center of gravity moves laterally by a distance equal to the space between the ankle joints. If the axis of the femur and tibia were collinear, then the lateral displacement would equal the distance between the hips. However, physiological genu valgus acts to minimize lateral displacement of the center of gravity during gait.

Because many common hip problems are associated with abnormal lower-limb biomechanics, an **assessment of gait** is an essential part of the clinical evaluation of hip complaints. In particular, the clinician should observe the following: 1) the relative duration of the stance phase for each leg, 2) the vertical motion of each shoulder, 3) the lateral motion of each shoulder, 4) anteroposterior shoulder movement, and 5) changes in pelvic obliquity during gait.

### Antalgic or Painful Gait

The hallmark of an antalgic gait is a shortened stance phase on the affected side, but as the patient tries to minimize both the duration and the magnitude of painful forces across the affected area, numerous compensatory patterns of gait may be observed. For example, patients with a painful great toe may walk on the lateral border of the foot or on the heel to remove force from the painful toe, and they are unlikely to exhibit the normal ankle plantar flexion and toe lift during preswing. A painful knee will tend to be kept in either flexion or extension, and heel strike is often modified by a short step onto a flat foot to keep the center of gravity over the knee and minimize the force acting across a distance behind or in front of the knee joint. Forces across the hip joint are particularly increased during stance phase because of the distance between the hip joint and the center of gravity. In addition to decreasing the duration of stance phase, patients with painful hip joint conditions often try to center the body over the affected hip joint, to minimize the joint reaction force. This involves a lateral movement of the trunk over the affected limb during stance. Thrusting the body weight over the hip joint minimizes pain by decreasing the force across the joint and by decreasing the necessity for the abductors—the gluteus medius and minimus, which may be involved with muscle spasm—to contract to maintain body balance; hence, it reduces pain and muscle spasm to some extent. This gait pattern is a combination of an antalgic gait and a compensated Trendelenburg gait. It is differentiated from an isolated Trendelenburg gait in the decreased stance phase observed in the combined gait pattern.

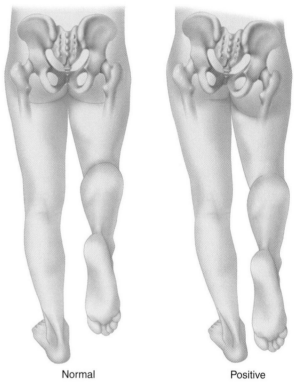

Normal                    Positive

**FIGURE 5-7    UNCOMPENSATED TRENDELENBURG SIGN.**

### Trendelenburg Sign and Gait

In 1895, Friedrich Trendelenburg described a clinical sign present in patients with **weak hip abductors** due to poliomyelitis or congenital hip dislocation. The Trendelenburg sign is observed by having the standing patient alternately raise each leg for at least 30 seconds. The examiner stands behind the patient and observes the pelvis. Normally, the pelvis rises up on the unsupported side due to contraction of the gluteus medius to maintain body balance, but the trunk should not swing over the stance leg by more than a few degrees. In a positive **uncompensated Trendelenburg sign,** the pelvis drops down toward the unsupported side. This indicates weakness of the abductor muscles of the planted leg (Figure 5-7). The dropping pelvis will be observed only if the patient is prevented from compensating for the weak abductor muscles by thrusting the body over the planted leg. If the patient must thrust the weight over the leg in stance phase

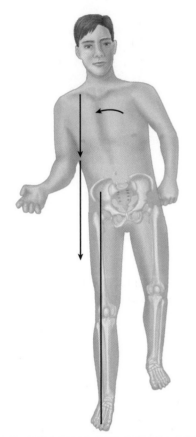

**FIGURE 5-8    COMPENSATED TRENDELENBURG SIGN OR GAIT.**

if the rib cage impinges on the pelvis in scoliosis. Severe knee varus deformity can cause a false-positive Trendelenburg sign or gait, because the hip abductors are poorly tensioned (i.e., the femur is always in relative abduction with respect to the pelvis).

### Leg-Length Discrepancy

To the patient, one leg may appear or feel relatively longer than the opposite leg for a number of reasons, including pelvic tilting due to spinal deformity (pelvis raised on the side of the shorter leg), fixed hip abduction, or fixed equinus of the ankle or foot. Conversely, a leg may feel short if there is a fixed hip adduction or a fixed flexion deformity of the hip or knee joint. With **true leg-length discrepancy**, the shoulder on the side of the short leg drops during that leg's stance phase. The knee of the longer leg may be held flexed when standing with the feet together, as the patient attempts to keep the pelvis level (see p. 56 for Leg-length Measurement).

### Astasia-Abasia

Although malingering is rarely encountered in normal medical practice, one does occasionally encounter a patient who is dealing with issues of secondary gain or a patient with psychological issues that result in abnormal gait patterns not based on any neuromuscular pathology. A malingering patient complaining of leg pain may demonstrate an increased duration of stance phase on the symptomatic leg, often accompanied by dramatic facial expressions of pain and the hands gripping the symptomatic leg, as the patient attempts to persuade the examiner how painful the leg really is. Others stand shaking and quivering, taking very small steps before collapsing into a nearby chair. It is important in these situations to be certain that there is no neurological problem that might account for the gait pattern. When recording findings that do not seem to be based on physiological pathology, it is best to simply report the incongruous findings (e.g., increased stance duration on the symptomatic side), rather than attaching a label to the patient such as "malingering patient" or functional overlay syndrome.

### Gluteus Maximus Gait

An individual with hip extensor weakness tends to thrust the pelvis forward while leaning back with the trunk and shoulders at heel strike. This passively extends the hip until the iliofemoral ligament becomes taut and stabilizes the lower extremity (see Figures 5-2 and 5-3). The center of gravity can then move forward over the planted leg without it collapsing.

### Drop-Foot Gait

Nerve injury to the peroneal division of the sciatic nerve results in weakness of the foot and ankle dorsiflexor muscles. With severe weakness of ankle dorsiflexion, the toes drag on the floor during swing phase, unless the patient lifts the foot higher than normal by exaggerated flexion of the hip and knee (**high-steppage gait**). The patient may also clear the ground by circumducting the leg out to the side during swing (**circumduction gait**). During heel strike, a weak tibialis anterior muscle cannot hold the foot, which slaps to the ground shortly after heel strike (**slap-foot gait**).

when lifting the opposite leg, this is considered a positive **compensated Trendelenburg sign** (Figure 5-8). Normally, a patient should be able to maintain the muscle force for at least 30 seconds. If the sign is initially negative (normal) but becomes positive within 30 seconds, this is known as a **delayed** (compensated or uncompensated) **Trendelenburg sign** and suggests muscle weakness or progressive pain inhibition of muscle contraction.

Assessment of the gait pattern may reveal a compensated Trendelenburg gait or, rarely, an uncompensated Trendelenburg gait. In an **uncompensated Trendelenburg gait**, the pelvis drops on the unsupported side during single-leg stance. This is rarely observed, as the patient would fall over without support on the opposite side with a cane or crutch. To compensate for the weak abductors, patients usually swing the body over the affected side, thus placing the center of gravity directly over the hip joint and eliminating the need for the abductors to contract. The appearance is similar to that of a **compensated Trendelenburg/antalgic gait** caused by hip joint pain with loading (described earlier), except that the stance phase duration is relatively normal in the absence of hip pain. A severe bilateral compensated Trendelenburg gait, or **waddling gait**, is characteristic of bilateral hip dislocation or weakness of the hip abductor muscles due to muscular dystrophy or poliomyelitis.

A positive Trendelenburg sign or gait may result from hip arthritis, an unstable hip, abductor muscle weakness due to poliomyelitis or muscular dystrophy, L5 nerve root impingement, and, indirectly, from loss of normal abductor muscle tension due to hip dislocation. The sign can also be positive

## PALPATION, LANDMARKS, AND SPECIFIC MANEUVERS

A number of structures and landmarks may occasionally be palpable in and around the hip joint. Many of these are not palpable routinely but can be examined when the clinical scenario is appropriate. Tendons and muscles should be carefully palpated if there is consideration of tendinitis or other pathology affecting these structures. Provocative tests involve active contraction of the musculotendinous unit against resistance and passive stretching in addition to direct palpation. These actions are likely to elicit pain of muscle inhibition when there is inflammation involving the tendon or the muscle.

### Is There Pathology of the Soft Tissues, Muscles, or Tendons?

*Femoral neurovascular structures.* The vascular status of both limbs should always be determined as part of a lower-extremity evaluation. A quick arterial screening test involves examining the quality of the distal skin and palpating the pedal pulses (dorsalis pedis and posterior tibial). If distal arterial circulation is intact, there is usually no proximal impediment to arterial flow, and a detailed examination of femoral and popliteal pulses may not be required. The femoral artery can be palpated just lateral to the midpoint of the inguinal ligament. The femoral vein lies immediately medial to the artery but usually cannot be palpated. The femoral nerve lies lateral to the artery, within the iliopsoas muscle sheath, and also cannot be palpated (Figure 5-9). Lymph nodes that drain the leg are located medial to the vein. Some nodes are normally palpable, but enlarged, painful nodes may indicate infection or other pathology.

*Sciatic nerve and adjacent structures.* With the patient in the lateral position, and the hip slightly flexed, the sciatic nerve may occasionally be palpable in thin individuals, just superior to a line connecting the ischial tuberosity and the greater trochanter, where the nerve lies on the obturator internus tendon and the quadratus femoris muscle. Tenderness in this area and just above it, in the greater sciatic notch region, may indicate sciatic nerve irritation or piriformis muscle spasm or inflammation. The piriformis muscle lies somewhat higher, above the line between the greater trochanter and the ischial tuberosity, but it usually cannot be palpated. The sciatic nerve typically exits through the greater sciatic notch just below the piriformis muscle, but it may penetrate the muscle or exit entirely above it (Figure 5-10).

*Bursae.* A *bursa* is a potential space with very little fluid that facilitates movement of adjacent soft tissues. It is usually not palpable unless bursitis with fluid distension has developed. Bursae are compressible but may be quite firm to palpation. A chronic bursitis may lead to loculation of the bursa, making it difficult to aspirate. There are a number of bursae about the hip joint. In **trochanteric bursitis,** there is tenderness over the greater trochanter and its posterolateral aspect, pain on resisted abduction and rotation, and, rarely, a local swelling. There is little or no pain on hip flexion or extension. **Iliopectineal bursitis** is associated with tenderness and sometimes a swelling just lateral to the femoral pulse in the groin, just below the inguinal ligament. The bursa becomes more tense and painful with hip extension. In **ischiogluteal bursitis** ("weaver's bottom"), there is tenderness and

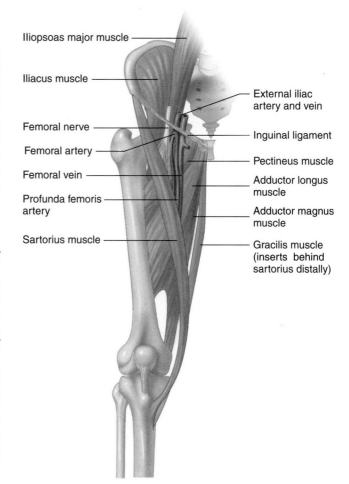

**FIGURE 5-9    THE FEMORAL TRIANGLE.**

Iliopsoas major muscle

Iliacus muscle

Femoral nerve

Femoral artery

Femoral vein

Profunda femoris artery

Sartorius muscle

External iliac artery and vein

Inguinal ligament

Pectineus muscle

Adductor longus muscle

Adductor magnus muscle

Gracilis muscle (inserts behind sartorius distally)

sometimes swelling over the ischial tuberosity. With hip flexion, the gluteus maximus moves off the tuberosity, and the bursa becomes more readily palpable and easier to inject. The differential diagnosis includes avulsion or tendinitis of the hamstrings, fracture, or osteitis of the tuberosity.

*Iliopsoas tendon pathology.* Iliopsoas dysfunction is a common source of complaints in athletes. The muscle belly of the iliacus can be palpated in a thin individual above the inguinal ligament. The iliopsoas tendon insertion into the lesser trochanter can be felt in some individuals with the hip in a relaxed position of 30° to 45° of flexion with slight external rotation and abduction. To palpate the lesser trochanter and distal iliopsoas tendon requires deep palpation in the femoral triangle just lateral to the femoral pulse.

A snapping sensation of the iliopsoas tendon may occur in dancers and other athletes. It can best be demonstrated by the patient recreating the maneuver that causes their symptoms but may be demonstrable in some cases by taking the hip from a flexed, abducted, and externally rotated position to an extended, adducted, and internally rotated position passively, or by asking the patient to do so actively. Passive stretch of an inflamed muscle or tendon will result in pain. The iliopsoas can be passively stretched by hip extension using a modified Thomas test, which we will discuss shortly.

Active muscle contraction is painful in the face of an inflamed musculotendinous unit. The iliopsoas can be

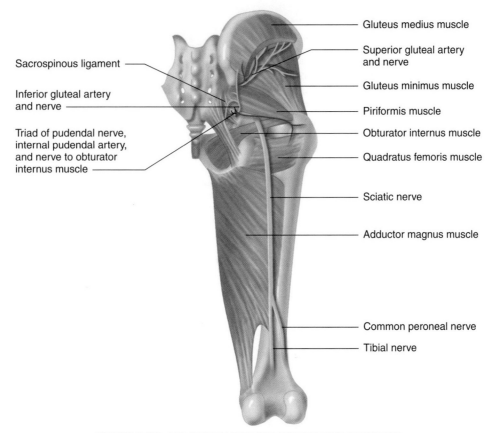

Sacrospinous ligament

Inferior gluteal artery and nerve

Triad of pudendal nerve, internal pudendal artery, and nerve to obturator internus muscle

Gluteus medius muscle

Superior gluteal artery and nerve

Gluteus minimus muscle

Piriformis muscle

Obturator internus muscle

Quadratus femoris muscle

Sciatic nerve

Adductor magnus muscle

Common peroneal nerve

Tibial nerve

**FIGURE 5-10    THE SCIATIC NERVE AND SURROUNDING STRUCTURES.**

isolated to some degree with the patient seated at 90° and the hip slightly externally rotated. The patient is then asked to flex the hip against resistance with the knee flexed or extended. Pain in the groin region may be due to inflammation along the iliopsoas or at its insertion into the lesser trochanter.

*Adductor tendon pathology.* The adductor longus and the gracilis tendons originate from the pubis just lateral to the pubic symphysis, where they may be palpated. They become prominent and can usually be visualized when the hip is abducted. A position of hip and knee flexion with hip abduction, while keeping the feet together in a frog-leg position on the examining table, may be more comfortable for the patient to maintain than abduction with the hip in extension. These tendons may be tender to palpation due to tendinitis or injury. Occasionally, the insertion of the tendon into bone may be traumatically avulsed, causing pain.

*Piriformis muscle pathology.* Piriformis syndrome is caused by piriformis muscle sprain or inflammation or by irritation or compression of the sciatic nerve as it passes the piriformis muscle posterior to the hip joint. A history of blunt, local trauma is common. Piriformis syndrome is associated with posterior hip pain produced by resisted external rotation of the hip with the hip and knee flexed at 90° (**Pace test**). Buttock pain—exacerbated by passive hip **F**lexion, **A**dduction, and **I**nternal **R**otation (**FAIR test**)—is also commonly present. In the **piriformis test**, the piriformis muscle is isolated by flexing the hip to approximately 60°, with comfortable knee flexion, in either the supine position or a lateral decubitus position. The examiner then passively stretches the piriformis muscle by bringing the knee into adduction

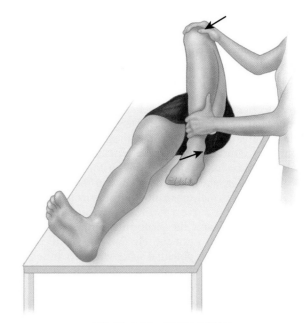

**FIGURE 5-11    PIRIFORMIS TEST.**

(Figure 5-11). Active abduction of the limb against resistance can also be tested. Pain results if the muscle or tendon is strained, and radicular pain may indicate sciatic nerve irritation at the level of the piriformis muscle.

A number of tests have been developed to evaluate specific conditions. These are applied as required based on the history of potential pathology.

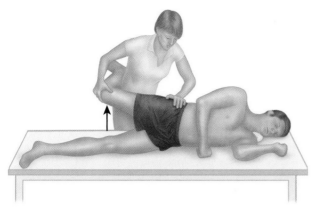

FIGURE 5-12    OBER TEST.

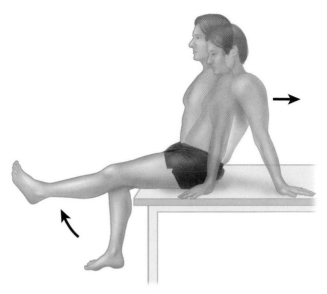

FIGURE 5-13    TRIPOD SIGN.

### Is There a Labral Tear of the Hip Joint?

Athletes complaining of groin pain should be evaluated for a possible tear of the hip joint labrum. A history of **clicking** in the hip joint is a highly sensitive symptom for this condition, but it is not specific. Stressing the labrum by internally rotating the flexed hip in adduction and applying axial compression may cause pain in the presence of a labral tear. A recent study found this maneuver to have a sensitivity of 75% for detecting labral tears but a specificity of only 43%. Apprehension and pain on external rotation of the extended hip may also be associated with a labral tear.

### Is the Iliotibial Band Tight?

With the patient in the lateral position, the uppermost hip being evaluated is abducted and extended, and the knee is flexed. On removal of the medial support, the normal hip passively adducts to allow contact of the knee with the examining table (**Ober test**). A tight iliotibial band prevents the hip from adducting passively (Figure 5-12). In complete deformity due to severe contraction of the iliotibial band, the hip is held flexed, abducted, and externally rotated; the knee is flexed with a genu valgus deformity; and pes equinovarus, unequal leg lengths, and compensatory lumbar lordosis are often present.

### Is There Iliotibial Snapping?

As noted above, one cause of so-called snapping hip involves the iliotibial band snapping over the greater trochanter. This occurs more commonly in a tight iliotibial band. The snapping is often best demonstrated by the patient. Often in single-leg stance, with the hip moved between flexion and extension, the addition of slight rotation in either direction will elicit the snap. The examiner may also ask the patient to lie in the lateral position, with the affected hip uppermost, and flex and extend the hip in both internal and external rotation to try and elicit the snapping.

### Is the Tensor Fascia Lata Muscle Tight?

Hip and knee flexion deformity may be caused by a tight tensor fascia lata muscle. Whether this is the case can be determined by the **Young test:** The hip is abducted to relax the tight tensor fascia lata muscle, and the hip and knee flexion deformity disappears if it was caused by a tight tensor fascia lata muscle.

### Are the Hamstring Muscles Tight?

The hamstring muscles cross both the hip and the knee joints. Hamstring muscle tension can be properly assessed only if hip flexion is normal, the hamstring muscles are relaxed (by flexing the knee), and there is no evidence of sciatic nerve root irritation. While the patient is sitting with hips and knees in 90° flexion, the knee is extended on the side being tested. If the hamstrings are tight on that side, the patient will lean back to extend the hip and avoid tension in the tight hamstring (**tripod sign** or **flipping sign**). To balance themselves on the examining table as they lean back, patients may place their arms behind them, creating a tripod to support the trunk (Figure 5-13).

### Is the Rectus Femoris Muscle Tight?

The rectus femoris muscle crosses both the hip and the knee joint. Muscle contracture can be demonstrated by noting movement at one joint as the muscle is stretched at the other. In the **Ely test,** the patient lies prone as the affected knee is flexed; a tight rectus muscle will cause the hip joint to flex, resulting in elevation of the affected buttock (Figure 5-14). Conversely, if the patient is supine, and the knee is flexed over the end of the examining table, the affected knee will extend as the hip joint is extended. (Hip extension is accomplished by flexing the opposite hip passively to flatten the lumbar lordosis, as in the Thomas test, and then pushing the affected hip into extension.)

### Is There Pathology Involving Bony Structures?

*Pubic rami.* Tenderness, and sometimes swelling, over the pubic rami and symphysis pubis occurs in **osteitis pubis.** It may also occur in spondyloarthropathies, trauma, and with pelvic infection, and the area should be palpated if this is suspected.

*Greater trochanters.* The greater trochanters are readily palpated in most individuals, in supine or standing position, by placing the extended fingers of both hands on the lateral aspect of each upper thigh and feeling gently from the buttock posteriorly to the thigh anteriorly, until the firm bony

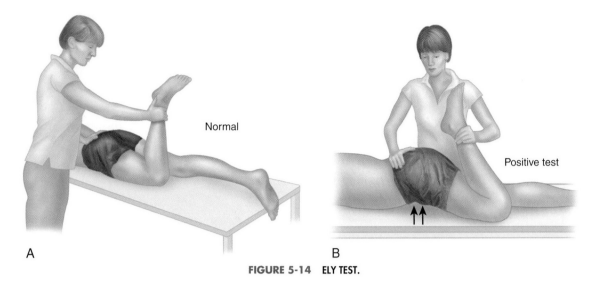

**FIGURE 5-14 ELY TEST.**

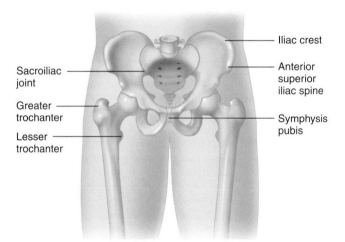

**FIGURE 5-15 BONY STRUCTURES OF THE HIP AND PELVIS: ANTERIOR ASPECT.**

prominence of the greater trochanter is detected. The superior and posterior aspect of the greater trochanter is usually the most readily palpable, and the superolateral area is generally the point of tenderness in trochanteric bursitis (Figure 5-15). Trochanteric bursitis is a common cause of hip pain, and palpation for tenderness in this area is usually part of a routine hip examination.

*Iliac crests and anterior and posterior superior iliac spines.* The iliac crest can be readily palpated in most individuals. The relative position of the two iliac crests in relation to the spine and the lower extremities is used to evaluate joint deformity and ROM. The most medial and distal point of the iliac crest is the **anterior superior iliac spine** (ASIS). This landmark is used as a reference point when measuring leg lengths, when assessing pelvic position in the measurement of hip ROM, and when evaluating pelvic obliquity. From behind, in the prone or standing patient, the PSIS can be palpated by following the iliac crest downward and posterior, until the most distal and medial point is reached (Figure 5-16). This landmark is used to further delineate the spatial orientation of the pelvis. It is also useful during surgery as a landmark for posterior approaches to the hip and acetabulum.

Palpation upward from the midline at the level of the posterior superior iliac spines reveals the S1 spinous process and, above it, the more prominent L5 spinous process.

*Ischial tuberosity.* The ischial tuberosity is most easily felt with the patient lying in the lateral decubitus position with the hip flexed. This area should be palpated if ischial bursitis is suspected.

## MEASURING LEG LENGTH

An **apparent or functional leg-length discrepancy** may be quantified by measuring from the xiphoid cartilage or umbilicus to the distal end of the medial malleolus of each ankle. Apparent leg-length discrepancy may be caused by pelvic obliquity or deformity, asymmetric hip or knee fixed flexion deformity, or a true difference in the lengths of the lower extremities (Figure 5-17). Measuring from a bony pelvic landmark, such as the ASIS, to the medial malleolus negates the effect of pelvic obliquity (see Figure 5-17) but may still be an inaccurate comparison of leg lengths if there is asymmetric fixed deformity in one hip or knee joint. Therefore, measurement of true limb lengths requires that any deformity on one side be replicated on the other before measuring. Sliding the tape up to the ASIS from below allows for easy identification of the landmark, even in a relatively heavy individual, and the distal end of the medial malleolus is readily identifiable.

**True leg-length discrepancy** may be caused by proximal displacement of the femur (collapse of the femoral head, hip dislocation) or by shortening of the lower-extremity long bones. A difference of less than 1.0 to 1.5 cm between the two legs can be normal and does not produce any significant functional problem. Shortening from the ASIS to the greater trochanter often indicates coxa vara, whereas shortening from the greater trochanter to the lateral knee joint line suggests shortening of the femoral shaft. Shortening of the tibial shaft is associated with shortening of the distance between the knee medial joint line and the medial malleolus. The length of the femur and tibia can be compared by direct measurement to the medial joint line of the knee or the medial femoral condyle, but direct observation with the hips and knees flexed and the heels placed a similar distance from the hips will uncover asymmetry below or above the knee

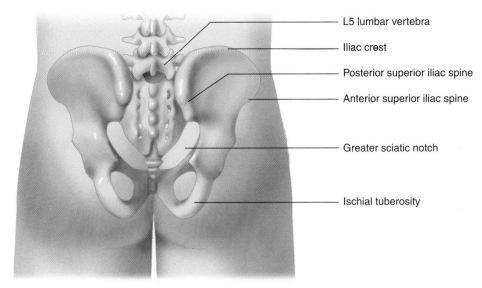

**FIGURE 5-16    BONY STRUCTURES OF THE PELVIS: POSTERIOR ASPECT.**

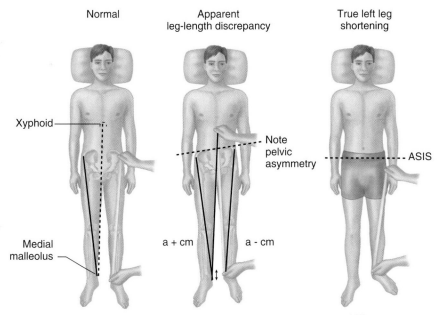

**FIGURE 5-17    LEG-LENGTH DISCREPANCY: NORMAL, APPARENT, AND TRUE MEASUREMENTS.** ASIS, anterior superior iliac spine.

joint, as manifested by the relative positions of the superior and anterior aspects of the knees (Figure 5-18).

The relationship between the greater trochanter and the pelvis can be used to determine whether the femur has migrated proximally by means of three tests:

1. *Nélaton's line:* The greater trochanter should lie at or below a line that connects the ASIS with the ischial tuberosity (Figure 5-19). Palpation of the greater trochanter above the line indicates coxa vara or a displaced hip.
2. *Bryant's triangle:* This test compares the relative height of the greater trochanter from one side to the other. With the patient lying supine, an imaginary perpendicular line is dropped from the ASIS to the examination table. A second line is projected up from the tip of the greater trochanter to meet the first line at a right

angle. This line is measured, and both sides are compared for coxa vara or displaced hip (Figure 5-20).

3. *Schoemaker's line:* Lines projected from the greater trochanter through the ASIS should meet above the umbilicus in the midline. Superior migration of one side causes the lines to meet on the opposite side. Bilateral proximal migration displaces the meeting point below the umbilicus.

## HIP RANGE OF MOTION

Hip ROM should be assessed actively and passively, paying particular attention to the location of any discomfort felt during mobility testing. In reality, passive testing is performed immediately after the patient has reached maximum active movement in the given direction, to maximize

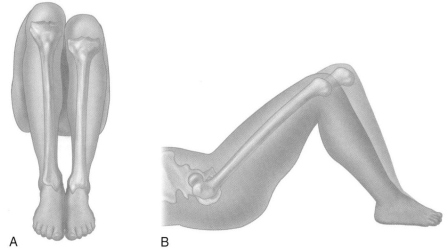

**FIGURE 5-18    LEG-LENGTH DISCREPANCY. A,** The tibia on the patient's left is shorter. **B,** The femur on the right is shorter.

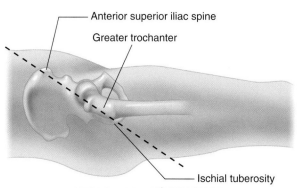

Anterior superior iliac spine
Greater trochanter
Ischial tuberosity

**FIGURE 5-19    NÉLATON'S LINE.**

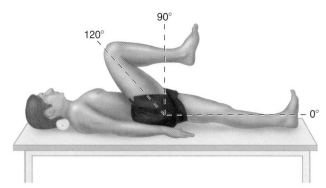

**FIGURE 5-21    HIP FLEXION.**

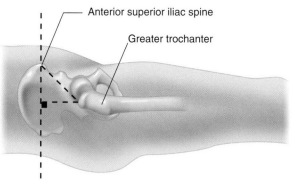

Anterior superior iliac spine
Greater trochanter

**FIGURE 5-20    BRYANT'S TRIANGLE.**

efficient flow of the examination. Normal ROM varies considerably but should not be painful. It is essential to compare the two sides, usually examining the more painful extremity last. After active and passive ROM have been assessed, the muscle strength of the movement is graded on a six-point scale, with values of 0, or no activity; 1, a flicker; 2, movement with gravity eliminated; 3, movement against gravity; 4, movement against resistance; and 5, normal muscle power.

### Hip Flexion

To test **active ROM,** the patient should be lying supine with legs extended and should be instructed to bring one knee up to the chest as far as possible; this will test hip flexion.

Extension is generally tested once the patient has either moved to lie on one side or is lying prone. In a prone position, the patient is instructed to move the leg up off the examination table. Care must be taken to make sure the patient is not extending at the lumbar spine to achieve this.

After the active flexion has been recorded, **passive ROM** should be tested. The patient should start by lying supine with the knee flexed, and the hip is flexed passively until a firm end point is reached (Figure 5-21). This may not occur until the knee touches the chest (about 120°), but other normal individuals may demonstrate only 100° of flexion. Even patients with a solid hip fusion may appear to have some hip flexion mobility due to pelvic rotation. To eliminate the possibility of misinterpreting pelvic rotation as hip flexion, the examiner should place a hand behind the upper pelvis and lower lumbar spine to monitor pelvic rotation. Once that firm end point has been palpated, the examiner should add a little extra stress in the direction being tested to test for **stress pain** that may be indicative of an actively inflamed joint.

Hip flexion power can be assessed with the patient supine or in a sitting position, beginning with the hip in approximately 90° of flexion. Although the rectus femoris also crosses the hip and knee joint, the **iliopsoas muscle** (L2, L3) is the main hip flexor. Because it inserts posteriorly into the lesser tuberosity of the femur, the iliopsoas can be isolated by externally rotating the hip during flexion strength testing.

## Hip Extension

**Hip extension** beyond neutral is limited in normal individuals to less than 20°. In the prone position, with the knee extended to slacken the rectus femoris muscle and the pelvis stabilized, the hip is actively and then passively extended. The point at which the pelvis begins to rotate represents the maximum amount of hip joint extension. The **gluteus maximus** (S1, S2, and also L5) is the principal hip extensor muscle, although there is some contribution from the hamstrings as well. Power can be tested in the prone position by applying pressure on the sacrum and asking the patient to lift the leg off the examining table. In the prone position, both hands can be applied on the distal limb to resist the powerful extension force, as the pelvis rests in a stable position on the examining table. Performing the test with the knee flexed isolates the gluteus maximus muscle. The patient with a fixed hip-flexion deformity may be unable to lift the leg off the table, depending on the degree of compensatory lumbar lordosis that can be generated. In this situation, the knee should be dropped off the side of the examining table, allowing the hip to flex so that strength can be tested. Alternatively, hip extensor strength can be tested in the supine position, beginning with the hip in flexion and resisting full hip extension with a hand under the heel.

*Thomas test for fixed flexion deformity.* When assessing hip ROM, it is essential to rule out a **fixed flexion deformity.** Such a deformity, which is common with hip joint arthritis, may be masked in the supine position due to an exaggerated lumbar lordosis that allows the legs to lie flat on the examining table. To assess for fixed hip-flexion deformity, the lumbar lordosis must be flattened completely by rotating the pelvis back, but care should be taken to avoid overrotating the pelvis and thereby overestimating the amount of deformity. The easiest way to rotate the pelvis is to use the opposite leg as a fulcrum. By passively bringing the opposite flexed hip and knee up toward the patient's chest, while feeling for flattening of the lumbar lordosis with the other hand behind the lower back, the correct pelvic position can readily be achieved. The patient may be asked to hold the flexed hip in this position with the hands placed around the knee to "hug" it toward the chest. Sometimes it is easier to flex both hips and knees until the lordosis is flattened. The hip to be tested is then extended until an end point is reached. If the femur can be dropped completely down to the examining table, no fixed flexion deformity of the hip is present, although extension may still be limited compared with the other side. The angle between the examining table and the femur of the limb being tested represents the degree of fixed flexion deformity in that hip joint (Figure 5-22). This maneuver was first described by Hugh Owen Thomas in the late 1870s and has become known as the **Thomas test.** It should be noted that a flexion deformity of the knee may masquerade as a fixed hip-flexion deformity, because it prevents the femur from lying flat on the table. In this circumstance, one can drop the lower leg of the side being tested off the side of the examining table. The angle between the table and the femur will then represent the magnitude of any fixed hip-flexion deformity. A fixed flexion deformity of the hip may be caused by capsular or muscle contracture or by joint deformity.

**Normal**

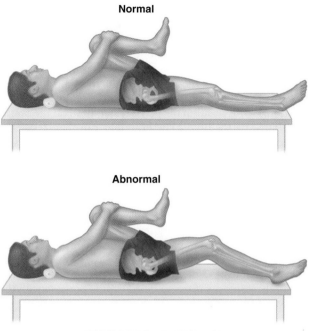

**Abnormal**

**FIGURE 5-22    THOMAS TEST.**

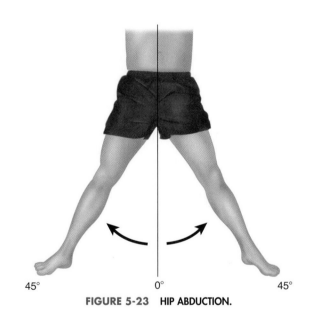

45°                                0°                                45°

**FIGURE 5-23    HIP ABDUCTION.**

## Abduction

Active and passive hip abduction can be measured in both flexion and extension. With the patient lying supine, the pelvis is stabilized by placing the examiner's hand on the opposite ASIS. The patient is instructed to abduct one leg at a time. Maximum abduction occurs at the point just before the ASIS begins to move, with any further movement representing pelvic tilt as opposed to hip joint motion (Figure 5-23). The same movement is then performed passively. Similarly, with the hip and knee in 90° of flexion, the knee is moved laterally toward the examining table. Again, lifting off of the opposite hemipelvis indicates the beginning of pelvic motion and the limit of hip joint abduction. Assessing abduction of both limbs simultaneously obviates the problem of having to stabilize the pelvis and can also reveal subtle differences between the two sides more readily than individual limb testing can. Normal hip abduction is about 45° in extension and 60° in flexion, although there is considerable interindividual variation. The gluteus medius (L5; also L4 and S1), along with the gluteus maximus (S1, S2) and the tensor fascia lata, which insert into the iliotibial band, represent the main hip abductors. Hip abduction power is most easily tested in the opposite lateral decubitus position. In this position the pelvis is stabilized on the examining table by the body. The examiner can then resist hip abduction either in full extension or in varying degrees of hip flexion.

### Adduction

When testing hip adduction, it is best to abduct the contralateral leg to provide space for the leg being evaluated, rather than crossing the legs during testing. Testing active adduction involves asking the patient to adduct one leg across the midline toward the resting leg. The pelvis should be stabilized. The same movement can then be performed passively. Again, this can be performed in the supine position with the hip extended or with the hip flexed. Normal hip adduction is up to 30°. The adductor muscles include adductor magnus, adductor brevis, adductor longus, pectineus, and gracilis (L3, L4, L5, S1). Adduction strength is best assessed by beginning with the hip in an abducted position and asking the patient to return it to the midline.

### Internal and External Rotation

Rotation can be assessed in either the prone position (Figure 5-24) or supine position, and it can be evaluated with either the hip in flexion or in extension. Active and passive internal and external rotation are generally performed as part of the same movement. With the patient in the supine position and the knee flexed to 90°, the patient is asked to rotate the raised foot down toward the resting foot while keeping the thigh flexed at 90°. This will test external rotation. Rotating the foot in the other direction will test internal rotation. This same movement is then performed passively. The examiner should make note of the relative position of each hemipelvis to detect pelvic rotation that could result in overestimation during rotation testing; however, it usually is not necessary to stabilize the pelvis manually. The main **external rotators** of the hip are the piriformis, obturator externus,

obturator internus, gemelli, and quadratus femoris muscles (L4, L5, S1). The iliopsoas and pectineus muscles are also weak external rotators. The normal range of external rotation is about 45°. **Internal hip rotation** is less powerful than external rotation. The normal range is about 40°. The gluteus medius, gluteus minimus, and tensor fascia lata are the main internal rotators (L4, L5, S1), with assistance from the semitendinosus and semimembranosus. Alternatives to testing this range-of-motion test **rotation in hip extension,** which can be accurately quantified with the patient prone. In the prone position, with the knees flexed to 90°, the angle between the tibia and an imaginary line perpendicular to the examining table can be used as a goniometer to measure internal and external hip rotation. It is important to remember that internal hip rotation involves rotation of the lower leg, rotating *away* from the midline, whereas external hip rotation involves rotation of the lower leg *toward* the midline. Rotation in hip extension with the patient supine, determined by rolling the leg medially and laterally, is less accurate and requires consideration of the transepicondylar femoral axis and the patella. Relying on the foot to demonstrate the amount of internal or external hip rotation can lead to errors.

For assessment of the strength of rotation with the hip extended, the patient lies prone with the knees 90° flexed. To test internal rotation, the patient is asked to move the foot from the midline *laterally* against the examiner's resistance. Similarly, external rotation of the hip is tested by asking the patient to move the foot *medially* against the examiner's resistance.

**Rotation in 90° of hip flexion** can be performed with the patient sitting, knees flexed over the edge of the examining table, or with the patient supine. In both positions, the tibia can be used as a goniometer relative to an imaginary midline bisecting the pelvis. To test rotation power in hip flexion, the supine or sitting patient begins with the hips and knees flexed to 90°. To test internal hip rotation, the patient is asked to move the foot from the midline *laterally* against the examiner's resistance. To test external hip rotation, the patient is asked to move the foot *medially* against resistance.

In general, at least 120° of hip flexion, 20° of abduction, and 20° of external rotation are required for performing activities of daily living. Hip joint stiffness makes it difficult for an individual to reach the toes for foot care (shoe tying requires about 120° flexion) or even to pull on socks and pants (requiring about 90° of hip flexion).

### Is the Sacroiliac Joint Painful?

There are many tests that attempt to stress the SI joints. The **FABER test** (Flexion, ABduction, and External Rotation) is also known as the **Patrick test,** but the **ankle-to-knee** or **heel-to-knee test** is the most common term for it. With the patient in the supine position, the affected hip is externally rotated with the knee flexed, so that the affected ankle can be placed on top of the opposite knee in a number-four position. Applying downward pressure to the affected knee stresses the hip joint and may cause typical hip pain. In the absence of hip pathology, when the pelvis is stabilized by applying pressure over the opposite iliac crest, the affected SI joint is stressed (Figure 5-25). Pain in the gluteal region of the stressed side is considered a positive test.

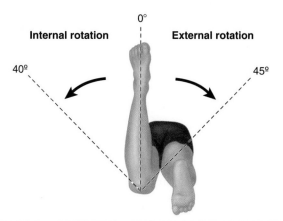

**Internal rotation**    0°    **External rotation**

40°                          45°

**FIGURE 5-24 HIP INTERNAL AND EXTERNAL ROTATION IN PRONE POSITION.**

The **Gillet test** evaluates the amount of SI motion in the coronal plane. With the patient standing, the examiner palpates the spinous process of S2 with one hand and the PSIS with the other. As the patient flexes the hip on the side being evaluated, the PSIS should normally move posteriorly and inferiorly with respect to S2. Absence of movement suggests sacroiliitis with fusion of the joint.

### What Is the Degree of Femoral Anteversion?

The femoral neck emerges at an angle from the femoral shaft relative to the femoral condyles distally. The angle changes from approximately 30° of anteversion in infants to 10° to 15° in adults. An assessment of femoral anteversion (forward torsion) and tibial torsion is essential when evaluating disorders of the lower extremities. Anteversion of the hip is the acute angle made by the femoral neck in relation to the femoral condyles. Excessive anteversion is more common in girls than in boys and can be associated with the patellae facing inward ("squinting patellae" and "toeing in").

Although a computed tomographic (CT) scan provides the most accurate method of measuring the degree of femoral anteversion, an approximation can be achieved by considering the position of the greater trochanter during hip rotation (**Craig test**). In a normal individual, the greater trochanter will be felt most prominently and directly lateral with 10° to 15° of internal hip joint rotation when the femoral neck is parallel to the floor. The degree of internal rotation required to bring the trochanter into this position can be noted in a prone patient with the knees flexed to 90°. The examiner places the greater trochanter into the most prominent position by rotating the hip. The angle between the leg and an imaginary line perpendicular to the floor from the knee denotes the degree of rotation required to achieve this position, which corresponds to the degree of femoral anteversion (Figure 5-26).

## Routine Hip Exam for the Chronic Painful Hip

Although there are many maneuvers and special tests that can be done during a hip examination, it is not generally necessary to perform all of these on each patient. Special tests are usually performed when a feature on the patient's history or physical exam has alerted the clinician that some other specific area should be tested to narrow down the problem. Although each clinician will develop a particular exam for their own purposes, a routine, screening hip exam should include the following:

Inspection with patient standing
    Gait
    Alignment and symmetry from the front, side, and back
Perform a Trendelenburg test (although this is a special test, it is best to do this before the patient moves to a supine position)
Inspection in supine position (skin condition, swelling, deformity, muscle wasting)
Palpation in supine position
Iliac crests
    Greater trochanter, bursa
    Anterior joint-line region for swelling or tenderness
Range of motion
    Flexion (active and passive)
    Internal and external rotation
    Adduction and abduction
    Thomas test for hip flexion contracture
    Extension

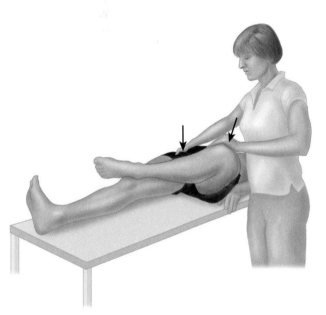

**FIGURE 5-25    FABER TEST.**

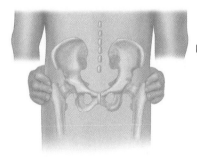

Palpate greater trochanter
parallel to table

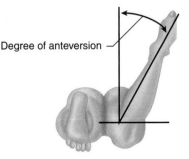

Degree of anteversion

**FIGURE 5-26    CRAIG TEST.**

Leg-length measurement
A routine hip exam should also include a screening knee and back examination (see Chapter 6)

## Aspiration and Joint Injection

### SACROILIAC JOINT

SI injections should be performed under fluoroscopic or CT guidance, because "blind" injections fail to enter the joint in almost 80% of cases. The SI joint is considered to be the source of pain if an injection of local anesthetic into the joint results in at least 75% pain relief. Although the joint space may accept up to 2.5 mL, excessive fluid injection may leak anteriorly and limit the diagnostic specificity of the injection by affecting other regional neural structures.

With the patient lying prone on a radiolucent table, the joint is approached from behind with a long spinal needle in the lower portion of the joint, just above the greater sciatic notch (Figure 5-27) and just below the PSIS. The needle is carefully advanced, slightly superiorly and laterally through the skin and subcutaneous tissue, at a 45° angle toward the affected SI joint. If bone is encountered, the needle is withdrawn and redirected more superiorly and laterally. After the needle enters the joint, aspiration and injection are performed.

### HIP JOINT

Hip joint aspiration and injection is best performed under fluoroscopic guidance. An arthrogram should always be performed to ascertain needle position within the joint capsule. An anterolateral, anterior, or medial approach can be used.

In the **anterolateral approach,** the needle is inserted along the femoral neck, beginning anterior and just inferior to the greater trochanter. The femoral neck is palpated with the needle until the capsule is entered, between 5 to 10 cm from the bone edge, depending on the size of the patient (Figure 5-28).

The hip joint lies approximately 2 to 3 cm lateral to the femoral artery, which can readily be palpated. In the **anterior approach,** the needle is inserted, under fluoroscopic guidance, approximately 2.5 cm lateral to the femoral artery and 2.5 cm distal to the inguinal ligament. The needle is advanced proximally and medially until the hip joint is entered, at 5 to 8 cm from the skin's surface (see Figure 5-28).

The **medial approach** is rarely used in practice. The leg must be flexed and abducted to permit ready palpation of the adductor longus muscle. The needle is inserted posterior to this muscle and advanced proximally and laterally from a starting point approximately 5 cm distal to the adductor muscle origin.

### BURSAE

#### Trochanteric Bursitis

With the patient lying on the nonpainful side, the greater trochanter is palpated to find the most tender area. The bursa is generally located in the posterolateral region. Once the area has been marked and prepared, a 25 gauge needle is inserted perpendicular to the skin, until the trochanter

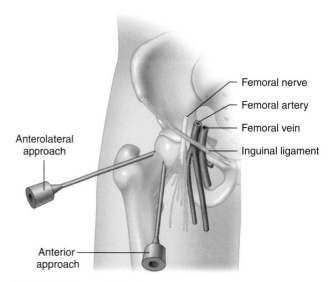

**FIGURE 5-28    HIP JOINT ASPIRATION: ANTERIOR AND ANTEROLATERAL APPROACHES.**

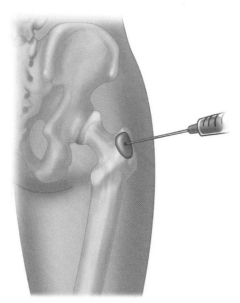

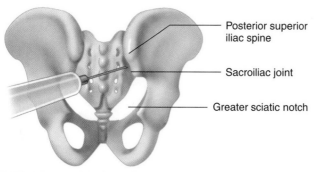

**FIGURE 5-27    ASPIRATION AND INJECTION OF THE SACROILIAC JOINT.**

**FIGURE 5-29    ASPIRATION AND INJECTION OF THE TROCHANTERIC BURSA.**

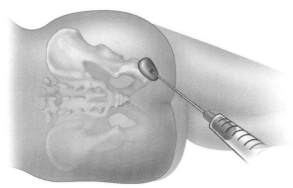

**FIGURE 5-30    ASPIRATION AND INJECTION OF THE ISCHIOGLUTEAL BURSA.**

lidocaine-corticosteroid mixture is injected, with care being taken to avoid needle-tip slippage off the tuberosity, which could injure the adjacent sciatic nerve (Figure 5-30).

is reached, and then withdrawn slightly before a lidocaine-corticosteroid mixture is injected in a fan-shaped fashion (Figure 5-29). In most patients, a 1½ inch needle is adequate to reach the trochanter. In patients with greater adiposity, a longer needle may be required.

## ISCHIOGLUTEAL BURSITIS

With the patient lying on the nonpainful side, hips and knees flexed, the site of greatest tenderness over the ischial tuberosity is identified. The needle is inserted at this site, and a

## SELECTED READINGS

Dreyfuss, P., Dreyer, S.J., Cole, A., et al., 2004. Sacroiliac joint pain. J. Am. Acad. Orthop. Surg. 12, 225–265.

Gross, J., Fetto, J., Rosen, E. (Eds.), 2002. Musculoskeletal Examination, second ed. Blackwell Publishing, Malden, MA.

Hardcastle, P., Nade, S., 1985. The significance of the Trendelenburg test. J. Bone Joint Surg. Br 67, 741–746.

Harris, N., Stanley, D. (Eds.), 2002. Advanced Examination Techniques in Orthopaedics, Cambridge University Press, London.

Magee, D.J., 2002. Orthopedic Physical Assessment, fourth ed. WB Saunders, Philadelphia.

Narvani, A.A., Tsiridis, E., Kendall, S., et al., 2003. A preliminary report on prevalence of acetabular labrum tears in sports patients with groin pain. Knee Surg. Sports Traumatol. Arthrosc. 11, 403–408.

Rosenberg, J.M., Quint, T.J., de Rosayro, M., 2000. Computerized tomographic localization of clinically guided sacroiliac joint injections. Clin. J. Pain 16, 18–21.

Slipman, C.W., Jackson, H.B., Lipetz, J.S., et al., 2000. Sacroiliac joint pain referral zones. Arch. Phys. Med. Rehabil. 81, 334–338.

Tile, M., Hefet, D.L., Kellam, J.F., 2003. Fractures of the Pelvis and Acetabulum, Third ed. Lippincott Williams & Wilkins, Philadelphia.

Vasudevan, P.N., Vaidyalingam, K.V., Nair, P.B., 1997. Can Trendelenburg's sign be positive if the hip is normal? J. Bone Joint Surg. Br. 79, 462–466.

# 6

# THE KNEE

Hans J. Kreder • Gillian A. Hawker

## Applied Anatomy

The knee is the largest synovial joint in the body. The knee joint is inherently unstable, because it is not constrained by the shape of its articulating bones. It consists of two tibiofemoral and one patellofemoral compartment. The **tibiofemoral articulation** is a condylar joint, whereas the **patellofemoral articulation** is a gliding joint (Figure 6-1). The **proximal tibiofibular joint** is a plain synovial articulation between the lateral tibial condyle and the fibular head. The tibiofibular joint capsule is much thicker anteriorly and is reinforced by the anterior and posterior tibiofibular ligaments. Slight movements occur at the joint with lower-limb rotation and with activities involving the ankle. The capsules and synovia of the knee and the proximal tibiofibular joints intercommunicate in about 10% of adults.

### JOINT STABILITY

The lack of congruity between the round femoral condyles and the flat tibial plateau requires that the tibiofemoral articulation be stabilized by soft-tissue structures to prevent joint dissociation. Various knee ligaments, the knee joint capsule, and the menisci act as **static stabilizers** that control knee motion, assisted by the surrounding muscles, which act as **dynamic stabilizers.** The capsule is reinforced by bands from the fascia lata, iliotibial tract, and tendons. Posteriorly the capsule is strengthened by the oblique popliteal and arcuate popliteal ligaments. The matching geometry of the femoral trochlea and the corresponding triangular undersurface of the patella contribute to patellofemoral joint stability. Patellar motion during knee flexion and extension is controlled by dynamic muscle-stabilizing forces, especially from the vastus medialis.

The exposed position of the knee joint and the lack of protective layers of fat and muscle make the knee highly susceptible to traumatic injuries. The location of the joint between two long bones also predisposes the articulation to maximum stresses.

### LOWER LIMB ALIGNMENT, PATELLOFEMORAL ARTICULATION, AND PATELLAR TRACKING

Normally, the center of the femoral head, the center of the knee joint, and the center of the ankle joint are aligned in the coronal plane (Figure 6-2). The adductor muscle mass normally produces the appearance of a relatively straight medial border from top to bottom in the lower extremity (Figure 6-3). Because the femoral neck offsets the femoral shaft away from the hip joint, the femoral shaft must meet the tibia at an angle (see Figure 6-2). This relationship has significant implications for the biomechanical functioning of the patellofemoral articulation. As the force of the quadriceps muscle contraction is transmitted through the tibial tubercle, at an angle to the quadriceps muscle pull, the patella experiences a laterally directed force. This force is resisted dynamically by the vastus medialis muscle (Figure 6-4), which is attached more distally to the patella than the vastus lateralis. The lateral femoral condyle projects more anteriorly than the medial condyle does, and this also helps to counteract lateral dislocation of the patella when the quadriceps contracts (see Figure 6-6A). The angle formed between the quadriceps muscle pull and the tibial shaft, known as the *quadriceps angle* or **Q angle** in a supine patient (see Figure 6-4), is normally between 8° and 14° in males and somewhat higher in females, although measurement error may be up to 5°, and there is disagreement regarding the upper limits of normal. The Q angle is measured between a line from the anterior superior iliac spine (ASIS) to the patellar midpoint and a line from the tibial tubercle through the patellar midpoint (see Figure 6-4). Weakness of the vastus medialis or a large Q angle is often associated with patellofemoral symptoms.

The undersurface of the patella is divided into a larger lateral and a smaller medial side by a vertical ridge. There are six paired facets—two each of a *superior, middle,* and *inferior*—and a seventh facet along the medial border. By holding the patellar tendon away from the axis of movement, at the femoral epicondyles, the patella provides leverage for the quadriceps to improve the efficiency of the last 30° of extension. During knee flexion, the patellar contact forces move upward on the undersurface of the patella, from the inferior to the superior facets.

When a person is standing erect, the knee is normally locked in extension, and no sustained quadriceps muscle contraction is required. Moreover, in full knee extension, the tibia rotates externally with respect to the femur, the so-called screw-home mechanism (Figure 6-5). Overextension and overrotation of the knee are prevented by the anterior cruciate, collateral, and oblique popliteal ligaments; an unexpected blow to the back of the knee causes the knee to buckle.

The knee is considered to be in the **close-packed position** during full extension, when the capsule and ligaments

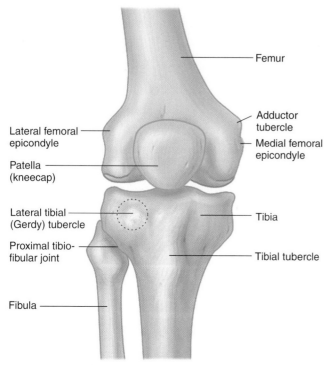

Femur

Adductor tubercle

Medial femoral epicondyle

Lateral femoral epicondyle

Patella (kneecap)

Lateral tibial (Gerdy) tubercle

Tibia

Proximal tibio-fibular joint

Tibial tubercle

Fibula

**FIGURE 6-1    THE BONES OF THE KNEE.**

are maximally taut and the articular surfaces are compressed and maximally congruent. The **open-packed position** occurs when the knee is flexed. The three lower-extremity joints—hip, knee, and ankle—can be considered a kinetic chain. **Open-chain** movements occur when the femur is relatively stable and the tibia moves freely, whereas **closed-chain** movements involve femoral movement over a fixed tibia. Open- and closed-chain movements can result in different types of sports injuries.

## KNEE LIGAMENTS AND SUPPORTING STRUCTURES

Although the main ligamentous structures about the knee (Figure 6-6) may be injured in isolation, knee-joint injuries often involve multiple ligaments, the joint capsule, and muscle insertions that act as static and dynamic knee-stabilizing structures (see Figure 6-5). In particular, the collateral and cruciate ligaments, posteromedial and posterolateral capsule, posterior oblique ligament, arcuate popliteus muscle complex, pes anserinus tendons, and iliotibial band represent the main **static knee stabilizers** (Figure 6-7). The hamstrings and quadriceps muscles serve as **dynamic knee stabilizers** by resisting anterior and posterior translation of the tibia on the femur, respectively. The fused tendons of the rectus femoris and vastis femoris (quadriceps tendon) insert into the upper patella, but some superficial fibers extend distally over the anterior patella to join the ligamentum patellae. Thinner bands from the sides of the patella attach to the anterior border of the tibial condyles to form the **medial and lateral patellar retinacula.** The gastrocnemius muscles make a more minor contribution to joint stability. The **fabella,** a sesamoid bone within the tendon of the lateral head of the gastrocnemius muscle, is present in approximately 10% to 20% of normal individuals. The

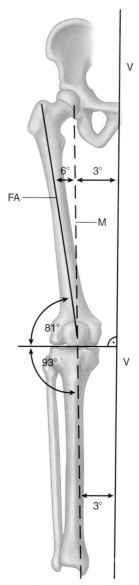

**FIGURE 6-2    LOWER-LIMB ALIGNMENT.** [From Gross J, Fetto J, and Rosen E ...ds.. *Musculoskeletal Examination*, 2nd ed. Malden, MA: Blackwell Publishing Company, 2002, page 293.)

fabella articulates on its anterior aspect with the posterior aspect of the lateral femoral condyle.

### Medial Collateral Ligament (MCL)

The medial (tibial) collateral ligament (MCL) consists of a deep and a superficial band. It attaches proximally to the medial femoral epicondyle immediately below the adductor tubercle and inserts distally into the medial tibial condyle (deep band) and into the medial surface of the tibia (superficial band or long band). The long, superficial band attaches to the tibia as a large fascial extension 7 to 10 cm below the joint line, deep to the pes anserinus tendons (Figure 6-8). The deep ligament band has attachments to the peripheral margin of the medial meniscus.

### Lateral Collateral Ligament (LCL)

The relatively small-diameter lateral (fibular) collateral ligament extends from the lateral femoral epicondyle proximally to attach onto the fibular head distally (Figure 6-9).

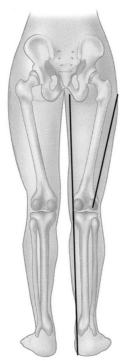

**FIGURE 6-3 LOWER-LIMB ALIGNMENT.** Straight medial border of the lower extremity.

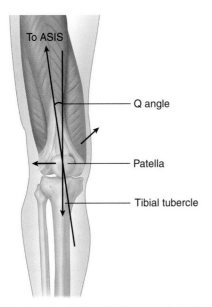

**FIGURE 6-4 MEASUREMENT OF THE Q ANGLE.**

### Anterior Cruciate Ligament (ACL)

The anterior and posterior cruciate ligaments, so named for the position of their attachment to the tibia, are situated centrally between the two tibiofemoral articulations (Figure 6-10). The cruciates provide a strong mechanical tie between the femur and the tibia, providing the main resistance to sagittal displacement; they also assist the collateral ligaments in resisting lateral bending of the joint. The **anterior cruciate ligament** (ACL) provides strong resistance to anterior displacement and excessive internal rotation of the tibia on the femur. The ACL attaches distally on the tibia

in a relatively large expanse just in front of and lateral to the tibial spine (intercondylar eminence). It spirals upward and laterally to attach onto the posteromedial corner of the lateral femoral condyle, posterior to the longitudinal axis of the femur. The ACL twists around the **posterior cruciate ligament (PCL)** with internal rotation of the tibia on the femur, and it may be injured either with excessive anterior translation of the tibia on the femur or with excessive internal tibial rotation. The ACL has been described as consisting of three distinct bundles; although this is a somewhat oversimplified representation of the ligament in vivo, it is nonetheless useful when dealing with partial ACL tears. The anteromedial fibers are taut in flexion, whereas the larger, posterolateral fibers are tight in extension. The intermediate fibers remain relatively taut throughout knee range of motion.

### Posterior Cruciate Ligament (PCL)

The tibial attachment of the PCL is extraarticular, extending down the back of the tibial plateau over 1 or 1.5 cm distal to the joint line (see Figure 6-6) and blending with the posterior horn of the lateral meniscus. On the femoral side, the ligament attaches onto the anterolateral aspect of the medial femoral condyle in the intercondylar notch on the opposite side of, and anterior to, the ACL (see Figure 6-10). The anterior fibers of the PCL are taut in flexion, whereas the posterior fibers are taut in extension.

During the **open-packed position** (knee flexion), the collateral and cruciate ligaments are lax, and flexion is not checked until the leg contacts the thigh. During the **close-packed position** (full extension), the cruciate ligaments become taut, preventing further extension. The collateral ligaments also prevent hyperextension as a result of their posterior attachment to the tibia and fibula.

### THE MENISCI

The menisci are semilunar structures, with a triangular cross-sectional geometry, that are situated around the periphery of the medial and lateral knee joint compartments (see Figure 6-10). They are composed of fibrocartilage and are attached to the edge of the medial and lateral tibial plateau beneath the femoral condyles. The peripheral border of the medial meniscus is firmly attached to the medial capsule in the deep portion of the MCL, whereas the free surface is invested by synovial membrane. The menisci cover about two thirds of the articular surface of the tibia. The menisci allow controlled rotatory movements during knee flexion and extension, and they attenuate forces during axial loading by increasing the contact surface area between the femur and the tibia (shock absorption). By deepening and improving joint congruity, the menisci also help to stabilize the knee. The menisci may have a role in joint nutrition by helping to distribute synovial fluid evenly to the surrounding articular cartilage of the femoral condyles.

### Medial Meniscus

The medial meniscus is C-shaped and has a larger radius than the lateral meniscus. The anterior horn of the medial meniscus is firmly attached to the tibia, just anterior to the ACL attachment. The posterior horn attaches adjacent to the PCL.

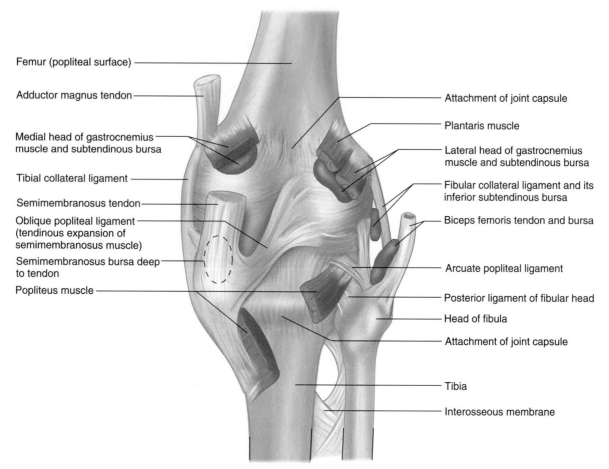

**FIGURE 6-5    POSTERIOR ASPECT OF THE KNEE.** Capsular, ligamentous, and muscular attachments.

### Lateral Meniscus

The lateral meniscus is more circular in shape, more mobile, and covers a larger portion of the articular surface than the medial meniscus. It is attached to the tibia between the tibial spines, between the tibial attachments of the medial meniscus. It is separated from the posterolateral joint capsule by the tendon of the popliteus muscle.

### The Synovial Membrane

The knee synovium is the largest in the body. It lines the inner surface of the capsule, suprapatellar pouch, cruciate ligaments, and free borders of the menisci. The suprapatellar pouch extends proximally about 6 cm above the patella.

## KNEE BURSAE

There are several bursae around the knee joint. These usually are not palpable unless they are inflamed (bursitis). The important ones are the following (see Figures 6-8 and 6-9):

1. Prepatellar bursa—overlies the lower half of the patella and the upper half of the patellar ligament
2. Superficial infrapatellar bursa—overlies the ligamentum patellae
3. Deep infrapatellar bursa—lies beneath the ligamentum patellae

4. Anserine bursa—located between the pes anserinus and the superficial part of the MCL over the anteromedial surface of the proximal tibia
5. Medial gastrocnemius-semimembranosus bursa

A popliteal cyst, also known as *Baker cyst*, is most commonly caused by a fluid-distended **medial gastrocnemius-semimembranosus bursa**, which may communicate with the knee through a posteromedial capsular defect in the medial joint compartment. The size of the cyst often varies over time and with knee position. A popliteal cyst can rarely be caused by a fluid-distended, communicating **popliteus bursa** (subpopliteal recess) through a defect in the posterior capsule of the lateral knee compartment.

### Blood and Nerve Supply

The knee derives its blood supply from a number of genicular branches from the femoral, profunda femoris, popliteal, and anterior tibial arteries. Its nerve supply is from the femoral, obturator, tibial, and common peroneal nerves.

### Knee Movements

The knee is not a true hinge joint, because the axis of movement is not a fixed one. Instead, the axis shifts forward during extension and backward during flexion. Also, the commencement of flexion and the end of extension are accompanied by rotatory movements. Therefore, movements of the knee from full flexion to full extension consist

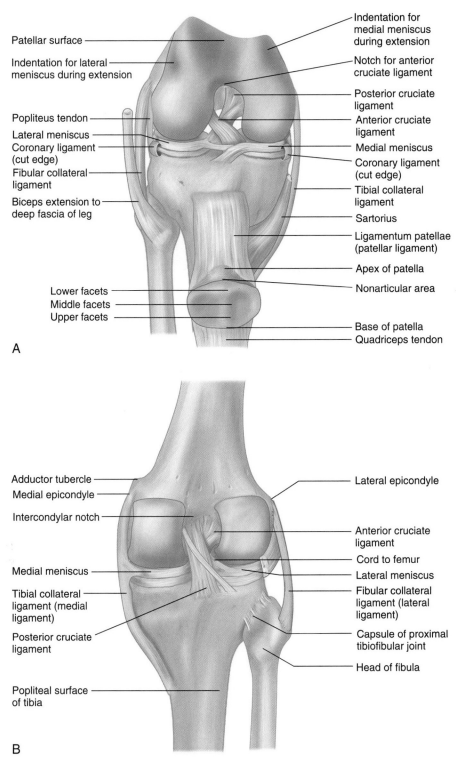

Patellar surface

Indentation for lateral
meniscus during extension

Popliteus tendon

Lateral meniscus

Coronary ligament
(cut edge)

Fibular collateral
ligament

Biceps extension to
deep fascia of leg

Lower facets

Middle facets

Upper facets

Indentation for
medial meniscus
during extension

Notch for anterior
cruciate ligament

Posterior cruciate
ligament

Anterior cruciate
ligament

Medial meniscus

Coronary ligament
(cut edge)

Tibial collateral
ligament

Sartorius

Ligamentum patellae
(patellar ligament)

Apex of patella

Nonarticular area

Base of patella

Quadriceps tendon

A

Adductor tubercle

Medial epicondyle

Intercondylar notch

Medial meniscus

Tibial collateral
ligament (medial
ligament)

Posterior cruciate
ligament

Popliteal surface
of tibia

Lateral epicondyle

Anterior cruciate
ligament

Cord to femur

Lateral meniscus

Fibular collateral
ligament (lateral
ligament)

Capsule of proximal
tibiofibular joint

Head of fibula

B

**FIGURE 6-6    LIGAMENTS OF THE KNEE. A,** Anterior aspect. **B,** Posterior aspect.

of three components: 1) a simple **rolling** movement of the tibia on the femur; 2) a **gliding** movement of the tibia on the femur superimposed on rolling, in which the axis of movement through the medial and lateral femoral condyle gradually shifts forward during extension (opposite to what occurs during flexion); and 3) a **rotatory** movement at the end of extension, consisting of external rotation of the tibia on the femur through contraction of the biceps femoris and tensor fascia lata. This rotary movement is referred to as the **locking**

**movement of the joint** or the **screw-home** movement. At the commencement of knee flexion, the converse occurs: the tibia internally rotates on the femur through contraction of the popliteus, semitendinosus, sartorius, gracilis, and semimembranosus, thereby "unlocking" the joint.

The screw-home position on full extension contributes significantly to knee stability, particularly when standing erect. It allows the patient to maintain knee extension over prolonged periods of standing without relying on continuous

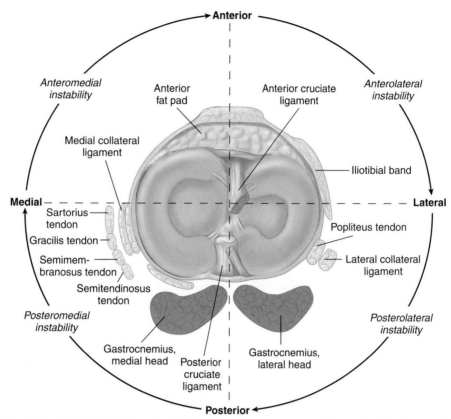

**FIGURE 6-7    STABILIZING LIGAMENTS AND MUSCLES OF THE KNEE.** (From Gross J, Fetto J, and Rosen E, eds. *Musculoskeletal Examination,* 2nd ed. Malden, MA: Blackwell Publishing Company, 2002, page 369.)

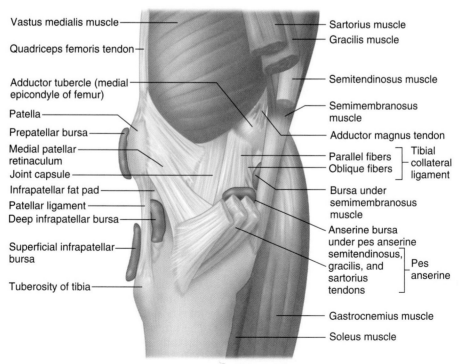

**FIGURE 6-8    THE KNEE: MEDIAL ASPECT.**

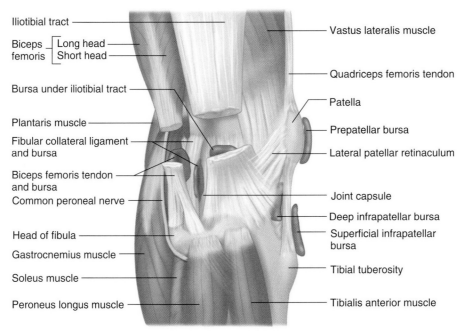

**FIGURE 6-9 THE KNEE: LATERAL ASPECT.**

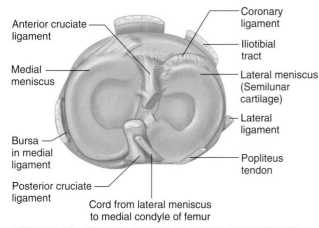

**FIGURE 6-10 THE KNEE: CRUCIATE LIGAMENTS AND THEIR TIBIAL ATTACHMENTS.**

quadriceps contraction; therefore, it is an energy-conserving mechanism. The presence of a knee flexion deformity abrogates this stabilizing mechanism, causing quadriceps muscle fatigue.

# Common Knee Disorders and Clinical Evaluation

## KNEE PAIN

If an injury is involved, it may be helpful to know the **direction of force** applied at impact and whether the knee was in the open- or close-packed position at the time. Knee pain is often diffuse and difficult to localize, but if the patient is able to delineate the **maximum area of pain,** this can be helpful in determining which underlying structure might be injured. Knee pain may be referred from hip pathology.

Occasionally, a patient is able to describe certain activities or movements that aggravate or alleviate the pain. For example, posteromedial knee-joint pain with squatting may be caused by a tear of the posterior horn of the medial meniscus. **Tendinitis pain** is often improved as a workout continues, whereas most other causes of pain usually increase with activity. Finally, the **pain character** may provide some clues as to the underlying pathology. Muscle pain is often felt as a deep, dull ache that is difficult to localize, whereas meniscus pain may be sharp, localized, and intermittent.

### Clicking, Snapping, and Clunking Noises and Sensations

Normal knees often make painless, high-pitched clicking sounds during squatting. Patients with arthritis or an inflamed synovium may note a crackling sound or sensation with knee movement. Low-pitched clunks may be caused by a loose body, a meniscus, or a cartilage fragment that is getting caught in the joint mechanism during movement. A patient may experience an audible snap or pop during rupture of a ligament or capsular structure or as a bone fractures.

### Swelling

Diffuse knee-joint swelling is a nonspecific symptom that suggests knee synovitis and joint effusion. Knee swelling that occurs immediately after an injury is often caused by bleeding into the joint from a ligament or capsular rupture or by an intraarticular fracture. Such bleeding is usually accompanied by bruising. Swelling that arises hours or days after an injury is more likely to be caused by inflammation rather than bleeding (e.g., acute synovitis). Swelling of the knee that occurs without injury suggests an inflammatory arthritis with synovitis and effusion.

### Heat and Redness

Swelling, heat, and redness are all signs of inflammation in the knee joint or periarticular tissues.

### Stiffness

Stiffness may accompany knee swelling, or it may be an independent symptom. With a large effusion, the knee is more comfortable in slight flexion, and patients have difficulty with both full extension and full flexion. They describe the knee as feeling "tight." Arthritis and periarticular contractures can cause decreased range of motion that is not due to fluid in the knee joint. A sense of stiffness in the morning is common with both rheumatoid arthritis and osteoarthritis.

### Deformity

Acute deformity after trauma suggests a major muscular, ligamentous, or bony injury that is accompanied by loss of integrity of the knee joint or the surrounding musculature sufficient to cause the deformity. For example, the patient may report noticing a lump at the lateral aspect of the knee that jumped back into place later on, suggesting a patellar dislocation that spontaneously reduced. The insidious onset of deformity often accompanies knee arthritis. Varus deformity of the knee is particularly common in medial compartment osteoarthritis.

### Giving Way and Instability

The knee collapses when the patient bears weight if the extensor mechanism is disrupted or inhibited by pain or muscle weakness. Patellofemoral problems often cause a sense of the knee's giving way, especially when descending stairs, because the quadriceps muscle is contracting eccentrically with controlled lengthening of the muscle. Disruption of the ACL can cause collapse of the knee with certain maneuvers that result in femoral translation into an abnormal position on the planted tibia.

### Pivoting

An ACL disruption allows the tibia to slide forward on the femur, especially on the lateral side of the knee. The patient may notice that this happens when the body is swung around to the outside of a planted leg during cutting sports. This movement rotates the femur around the tibia, and, because of the incompetent ACL, the femur rides back excessively on the lateral side. Patients often describe what happens by using their fists to indicate how the knee pivots. Pivoting is often accompanied by painful collapse as the knee joint gives way.

### Locking

True locking of the knee refers to sudden or recurrent inability to flex or to extend the knee. It can occur because of a mechanical block to knee-joint motion, such as a loose body, meniscus flap, cruciate ligament stump, cartilage flap, or scar tissue that interferes with knee flexion or extension by its interposition between the joint surfaces. True locking must be distinguished from **pseudolocking,** which is caused by knee-joint stiffness or lack of movement due to pain inhibition, as opposed to a mechanical block. Asking the patient whether the knee "jams up" or "gets stuck" because something seems to be caught in it may be helpful in differentiating true locking from pseudolocking.

### INFLAMMATORY ARTHRITIS AND OSTEOARTHRITIS

Symptoms of arthritis include pain, swelling, stiffness, crepitus, and, in the late stages, deformity and instability. Physical findings include disuse atrophy of the vastus medialis, joint tenderness, joint effusion, joint instability, and decreased range of motion. There may be similar changes found in other joints, the distribution of which may provide clues for the diagnosis of inflammatory arthritis. For example, rheumatoid arthritis generally produces symmetrical swelling of small and large joints.

### LIGAMENTOUS INJURY

Ligamentous injury should be ruled out in the assessment of any patient who presents with knee pain after an acute injury. The direction of impact should be sought if possible, considering that the ligaments opposite to the impact may have been ruptured. Whereas complete ligament disruption is associated with gross instability, a grade 1 tear may be painful in the absence of instability on history or physical examination.

In the acutely injured patient, the Lachman test is particularly useful, because it has both a high positive and a high negative predictive value for **ACL injury diagnosis** (Table 6-1). The pivot shift test is very useful, if it is positive; but injuries can be missed, especially in the acute situation, when a patient is apprehensive and in muscle spasm. The anterior drawer test is less accurate than the Lachman test. For the **diagnosis of PCL injuries,** the posterior sag, posterior drawer, and quadriceps active tests are all useful, especially for diagnosis of chronic injuries (see Table 6-1). Isolated ligament ruptures are relatively rare, and combined injuries with capsular tears, tibial plateau fractures, or meniscal injuries are more common.

### FRACTURE

Significant traumatic fractures of the articular surface or metaphyseal region are obvious by the sudden loss of function with accompanying swelling and deformity. However, some types of tibial plateau fractures are quite subtle and easily missed. A lateral blow may result in a compression fracture of the lateral plateau in association with an MCL injury. The patient may be able to walk, and the MCL injury may distract the examiner from thoroughly assessing the lateral plateau. Moreover, because the lateral femoral condyle impacts into the depressed tibial plateau, the examiner may mistakenly interpret valgus instability as MCL instability. It is essential to consider the neutral starting position when assessing instability, which should be tested in full extension, and in various degrees of flexion, and compared with the other side. An anterior tibial plateau fracture can cause instability in full extension in the absence of collateral or cruciate ligament damage. A posterior depressed fracture of the tibial plateau may demonstrate no instability in extension but marked instability in flexion. If such injuries are neglected, the patient may be unable to get up from a chair or use stairs without buckling of the knee, because the knee is loaded in flexion.

### MENISCUS INJURY

A history of an injury with subsequent locking, clunking, and localized pain to the joint line is a classic for a meniscus tear. The accuracy of physical examination maneuvers in correctly diagnosing meniscus pathology is low according to the published literature (see Table 6-1). Unquestionably, the evaluation of meniscus pathology requires attention to detail and skill that can be acquired only with experience. Careful application

TABLE 6-1

## ACCURACY OF DIAGNOSTIC TESTS USED IN KNEE EXAMINATION

| | Test Sensitivity | Specificity | LIKELIHOOD RATIO | |
| | | | Positive | Negative |
|---|---|---|---|---|
| **ACL tear** | | | | |
| Anterior drawer test (awake) | 0.22–0.41 | 0.78–0.99 | 3.8 | 0.30 |
| Anterior drawer test (general anesthesia) | 0.80–0.91 | NA | | |
| Lachman test | 0.86 | 0.91 | 42.0 | 0.1 |
| Pivot shift test | 0.32 | 0.98 | 15.08 | 0.7 |
| **PCL tear** | | | | |
| Posterior drawer test (acute) | 0.51–0.86 | NA | NA | NA |
| Posterior drawer test (chronic) | 0.90 | 0.99 | 90 | 0.1 |
| Quadriceps active test (chronic) | 0.54 | 0.97 | 18 | 0.5 |
| Posterior sag (chronic) | 0.79 | 0.99 | 79 | 0.2 |
| **Patella** | | | | |
| Patellar apprehension sign | 0.39 | NA | NA | NA |
| MPAT | 1.00 | 0.88 | NA | NA |
| **Meniscus** | | | | |
| Joint-line tenderness | 0.79 | 0.15 | 0.9 | 1.1 |
| McMurray test | — | 0.59 | 1.3 (NS) | 0.8 (NS) |
| Medial lateral grind test | 0.69 | 0.86 | 4.8 (NS) | 0.4 |

ACL, anterior cruciate ligament; PCL, posterior cruciate ligament; NA, not applicable; NS, not statistically significant
(From Gross J, Fetto J, Rosen E: *Musculoskeletal Examination*, 2nd ed. Malden, MA: Blackwell Publishing, 2002; Harris N: *Advanced Examination Techniques in Orthopaedics.* Greenwich Medical Media, 2003; Malanga GA, Andrus S, Nadler SF, McLean J: Physical examination of the knee: A review of the original test description and scientific validity of common orthopedic tests. *Arch. Phys. Med. Rehabil.* 2003;84:592–603.)

of the meniscus tests described earlier, in conjunction with a detailed history, should allow the examiner to limit the use of magnetic resonance imaging (MRI) studies to those cases in which significant uncertainty remains after the clinical evaluation. An acutely injured knee may be exceedingly difficult to examine for a meniscus injury. For example, it is impossible to perform a McMurray test unless the knee can be flexed to at least 90°. A repeat examination 1 or 2 weeks after the acute injury is often very helpful in establishing the correct diagnosis.

## REPETITIVE STRAIN AND OVERUSE INJURIES

A number of overuse injuries, resulting from repetitive activities that place stress on the knee, have been described. **Runner's knee** often refers to patellofemoral syndrome caused by abnormal patellar tracking, but it may also denote lateral knee pain resulting from iliotibial band friction syndrome. **Jumper's knee** in adults refers to proximal patellar tendinitis, whereas in adolescents it denotes either distal patellar tendinitis (Larson-Johansson disease) or traction epiphysitis (Osgood-Schlatter disease). **Swimmer's knee** or **breaststroker's knee** denotes anserine bursitis. **Carpet layer's, miner's,** or **housemaid's knee** refers to traumatic prepatellar bursitis. **Gamekeeper's knee** describes medial gastrocnemius-semimembranosus bursitis caused by excessive knee flexion.

## CONSIDERATIONS IN PATIENTS AFTER TOTAL KNEE REPLACEMENT

### Safety Considerations

In complex knee revision surgery, the extensor mechanism or the collateral ligaments may be compromised. The examiner should avoid undue force when examining for passive range of motion or when testing the integrity of the ligaments in these situations. Certain types of knee implants may click, especially during testing for stability in flexion, as the artificial components move apart a few degrees and then back together. This usually is not a sign of pathology. Some numbness around the incision site is common, but a painful trigger point near the incision may indicate the presence of a neuroma.

### Pain after Total Knee Arthroplasty

*Mechanical failure.* **Knee dislocation** and **periprosthetic distal femoral fractures** or **proximal tibial fractures** generally result in severe functional impairment, usually with complete inability to walk, severe pain, and an often characteristic deformity. Knee dislocation is extremely rare early on, but it can occur after significant wear of the components has rendered the interface unstable or with subsidence or loosening of one or more implant components. A thorough neurovascular examination is essential in these situations, considering the proximity of the vascular trifurcation and the common peroneal nerve. The patellofemoral joint should be evaluated after total knee replacement surgery for possible **patellar maltracking** related to implant position, quadriceps muscle imbalance, and soft-tissue contractures. This entails an assessment of alignment that includes the Q angle, the relative height of the patella, and quadriceps muscle bulk and strength, as well as a dynamic impression of patellar tracking as the patient flexes and extends the knee. Problems with patellofemoral function may severely impair walking ability, because the knee gives way during loading.

### Neurovascular Pain and Dysfunction

The **common peroneal nerve** is particularly at risk for injury when a preoperative fixed valgus deformity is corrected at the time of knee replacement, resulting in lengthening of the lateral side of the knee and stretching of the peroneal nerve. Complaints of pain and paresthesia should be evaluated with a complete neurological examination. The most obvious motor abnormality with complete loss of common peroneal nerve function is a dense foot drop.

### Deep Vein Thrombosis

Patients are at significant risk for deep vein thrombosis (DVT) after total knee replacement surgery. Most surgeons use thromboprophylaxis for a variable period after surgery, and the patient should be questioned about the specifics of this treatment. The clinician should have a high index of suspicion for the possibility of DVT, especially if the patient has gone 8 to 12 weeks since the surgery and is no longer receiving thromboprophylaxis. Physical examination is poor at determining whether DVT is present, and diagnostic tests, such as ultrasound or venography, should be used liberally if DVT is suspected.

### Implant Loosening and Infection

Mechanical loosening of the implant–bone interface may be associated with pain. Important causes of loosening include trauma, osteolysis due to implant wear, and infection. The examiner should inquire about recent falls or other **injuries** and the relationship of these events to the onset of pain. Information regarding how long the knee replacement has been in situ can provide clues regarding the possibility of **implant wear**. Finally, potential sources of **infection** should be sought. Low-grade infections may go undetected for many months before implant loosening or systemic manifestations are noted. Typically, pain due to infection is always present and is not relieved with rest, whereas mechanical loosening may result in intermittent pain, usually with activity. If infection is suspected, knee aspiration and fluid culture are indicated. Early postoperative infection can sometimes be managed with debridement with successful retention of the implants.

### Other Causes

Bursitis around the knee can be a potential cause of knee pain after prosthetic implantation. For example, medial overhang of the tibial component may cause pes anserine bursitis. Referred knee pain from the hip joint or lumbar spine is another potential source of pain.

## Physical Examination

It is essential to fully expose both legs when evaluating knee complaints. This requires the patient to undress down to short underwear or to use athletic shorts and appropriate drapes. A patient with an acute knee injury may be more comfortable in the open-packed position with the knee slightly flexed and a supporting pillow behind the joint. It is essential to examine both the knees and the lower limbs, the asymptomatic knee first, when assessing unilateral or bilateral knee complaints.

An experienced examiner evaluates the knee joint in a systematic but focused manner by first performing those maneuvers and tests that are likely to have the highest positive or negative yield with respect to the specific differential diagnoses being considered. Moreover, for patient comfort, and to make the examination flow more smoothly, those tests that can be done with the patient in the supine position and the knee in extension are carried out before other tests (i.e., those that require knee flexion or a prone or standing position).

Throughout the history taking and physical examination, the clinician seeks to refine and validate hypotheses about the underlying pathology and synthesize the available information into a brief but meaningful differential diagnosis. For example, is this referred pain, or is there evidence of knee-related problems? The presence of a joint effusion indicates underlying knee pathology. Is the joint swelling caused by an acute ligamentous disruption, a meniscus tear, or an arthritic condition? As with all lower-extremity evaluations, it is important to perform a screening evaluation of the spine and neurovascular structures, as well as the hip and ankle joints, bilateral leg lengths, and lower-limb angular and rotational alignment. In the case of knee swelling in the absence of a history of injury, it is also essential to examine the upper extremity for evidence of joint inflammation suggesting arthritis. Furthermore, inflammatory arthritis can be associated with a number of extraarticular findings, such as rash or any changes detected in lung or heart examination. Thus, a careful general physical examination is generally warranted in the setting of possible inflammatory arthritis.

Although it may be useful to consider inspection, palpation, and movement separately when teaching physical examination techniques, it is more helpful to consider what information is actually being sought and how a specific maneuver may help to provide that information. Thus an experienced examiner performs an examination with questions in mind that the examination is meant to answer, rather than artificially performing a full-knee palpation examination, followed by a test of movements and other specific maneuvers.

## INSPECTION

Inspection begins with an evaluation of the patient as a whole. Are there clues as to the presence of a chronic systemic condition, such as rheumatoid arthritis? Is the patient generally fit in appearance, or are they above ideal body weight for height? Localized evaluation involves an assessment of the skin, subcutaneous tissue, muscles, and bony landmarks. Skin incisions or scars should be explained by the patient, and any relationship to the current symptoms should be explored. Psoriatic skin lesions and nail changes raise the possibility of psoriatic arthritis. Skin discoloration, ulceration, and distal hair loss may be associated with vascular insufficiency. Unilateral knee swelling may be a sign of joint effusion or bursitis. Bony enlargement along the joint margins may signify osteophyte formation in osteoarthritis. Wasting of the distal quadriceps muscle, especially the vastus medialis, is consistent with disuse atrophy. Normally, the vastus medialis produces an obvious muscle bulge in the region adjacent to the upper portion of the patella; a hollow in this region suggests disuse atrophy. An effusion usually produces a swelling more distally on the medial aspect of the knee.

The integrity of the extensor mechanism of the knee can be tested by asking the supine patient to raise the leg off the examining table. In the absence of severe pain, inability to

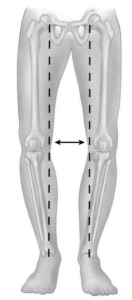

**FIGURE 6-11    GENU VARUM.**

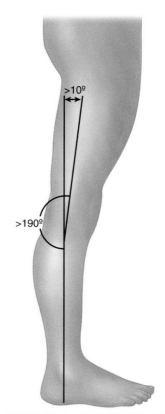

**FIGURE 6-13    GENU RECURVATUM.**

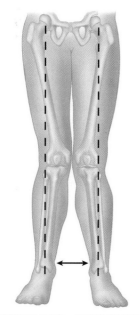

**FIGURE 6-12    GENU VALGUM.**

raise the heel off the table suggests hip joint pathology or loss of extensor function due to quadriceps weakness, rupture of the quadriceps tendon, fracture of the patella, or rupture of the patellar tendon. An individual with a large knee-joint effusion or a meniscus tear may not be able to fully extend the knee. In the frontal view, the patella should lie in between the two femoral epicondyles and in the same plane as the center of the femoral head and the center of the ankle joint.

### Genu Varum and Genu Valgum

Normally, the center of the knee joint lies on a line that connects the center of the hip and the center of the ankle joint (see Figure 6-2). In an individual with **genu varum,** or **bowleg deformity,** the center of the knee joint falls lateral to the axis connecting the centers of the hip and ankle

joints (Figure 6-11). Although accurate assessment of bony alignment requires radiographic imaging, a patient with more than 3 cm of space between the medial femoral condyles when standing with the feet together probably has genu varum. Conversely, **genu valgum,** or **knock-knee deformity,** occurs when the center of the knee joint is medial to the biomechanical axis of the lower extremity (Figure 6-12). Clinically, an individual with more than 3 cm between the medial malleoli likely has genu valgum. Inspection for varus or valgus misalignment is best performed with the knee in a weight-bearing (standing) position.

### Genu Recurvatum and Genu Procurvatum

When the knee is examined from the side, the patient should be able to fully straighten it. A few degrees of hyperextension can be normal, especially in patients with generalized ligamentous laxity; but more than 10° of hyperextension, or **genu recurvatum** ("back knees"), generally indicates pathology such as hypermobility syndrome or a cruciate ligament laxity or injury (Figure 6-13). A fixed flexion deformity (**genu procurvatum**) or the inability to achieve full extension is always pathological and may be caused by arthritis, a large joint effusion, or a mechanical block to extension resulting from a meniscus tear or loose body.

### Squinting and Frogeye Patellae

**Squinting patellae,** patellae that are facing toward each other when the patient walks toward the examiner with feet pointing forward, suggest an internal rotational deformity of the femur or an external rotational deformity of the tibia (Figure 6-14). External femoral rotation or internal tibial

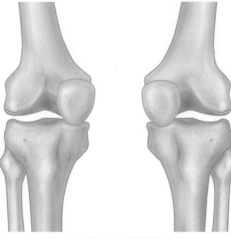

FIGURE 6-14    SQUINTING PATELLAE.

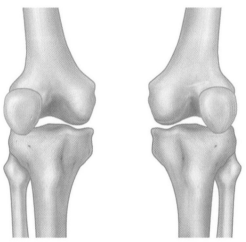

FIGURE 6-15    FROGEYE PATELLAE.

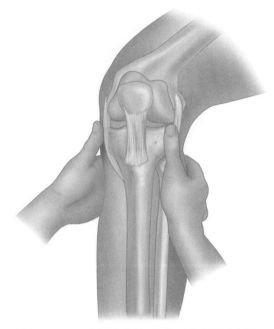

FIGURE 6-16    PALPATION OF THE MEDIAL AND LATERAL TIBIAL PLATEAUS AND JOINT LINES.

rotation gives the appearance of patellae that face away from each other (**frogeye patellae;** Figure 6-15).

### Knee Swelling

A diffuse, generalized knee swelling usually indicates either a joint effusion or a diffuse inflammatory synovitis with synovial thickening. By contrast, an asymmetric, localized swelling often suggests a bursitis or tendon lesion. Medial swelling can be caused by a small knee-joint effusion. A popliteal cyst located behind the medial compartment of the knee is often caused by a distended, communicating medial gastrocnemius-semimembranosus bursa. Less commonly, a cyst behind the lateral compartment suggests a swollen, communicating popliteus bursa. In the setting of inflammation, the skin overlying the knee may appear erythematous.

## PALPATION AND SPECIFIC MANEUVERS

Many acute and chronic knee problems are associated with knee-joint inflammation and knee-joint effusion. Determining whether evidence of such pathology exists is a good place to begin the general physical examination of the knee joint. The knee examination should consider the following structures: soft tissues (muscles, tendons, and bursae); bone structures, including consideration of bone alignment; the collateral and cruciate ligaments; the menisci; and the medial, lateral, and patellofemoral knee articulations.

### What Is the Vascular Status of the Limb?

It is essential to assess the vascular status of both lower extremities as part of a knee evaluation. Some examiners are in the habit of performing the vascular examination as the very first or very last part of the overall evaluation to ensure that it is not missed inadvertently. In addition to inspecting for vascular skin compromise, palpation of the pedal pulses (dorsalis pedis and posterior tibial) can be used as a quick screening test. If the distal vascular status is intact, this suggests that there is no compromise to the arterial circulation of the entire extremity. In the absence of pedal pulses, palpation of the popliteal and femoral pulses is required. Circulatory problems are a potential cause of leg pain and may also increase the risk of surgical complications, if an operation is required.

### Is the Knee Joint Inflamed?

The normal knee should be slightly cooler to the touch than the adjacent anterior thigh, which is surrounded by a well-perfused muscle layer. A knee that feels as warm as or warmer than the thigh is likely to be inflamed. Other signs of knee synovitis include redness, swelling, and a joint effusion. Synovitis of the knee is characterized by synovial thickening and diffuse joint-line tenderness, both along the medial and lateral compartments. The synovium is best palpated along the joint line with the knee 90° flexed. Normally, the synovial membrane is quite thin and difficult to palpate. Chronic synovitis, caused by rheumatoid or other inflammatory arthritis, is often associated with significant synovial thickening, with more soft tissue intervening between the palpating thumbs and the joint line (Figure 6-16).

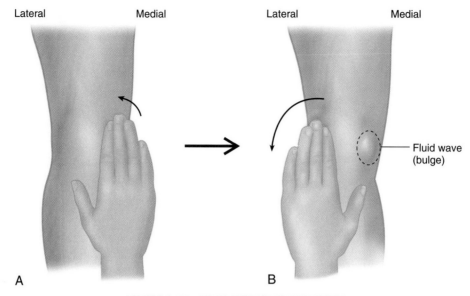

Lateral          Medial          Lateral          Medial

Fluid wave
(bulge)

A                          B

**FIGURE 6-17    BULGE SIGN FOR KNEE EFFUSION.**

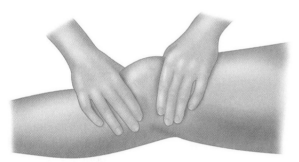

**FIGURE 6-18    BALLOON TEST.**

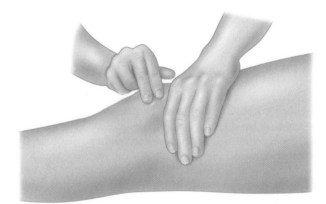

**FIGURE 6-19    PATELLAR TAP TEST FOR KNEE EFFUSION.**

## Is There Fluid in the Knee Joint?

Rapid fluid accumulation in the knee after an injury suggests that bleeding from a vascular structure, such as the ACL, has occurred. Osteoarthritic, inflammatory, or infectious conditions cause more gradual accumulation of a knee effusion.

*Bulge sign.* In the **brush, stroke,** or **wipe test,** fluid is pushed up into the suprapatellar pouch by sliding the hand from the distal aspect to the proximal along the medial aspect of the knee joint with the patient in the supine position and the knee relaxed in extension. The fluid is then milked back down by sliding the hand from the superior aspect to the inferior along the lateral aspect of the knee (Figure 6-17). A medial fluid bulge indicates free fluid within the knee joint (**bulge sign**). The test can be used to demonstrate small to moderate effusions (less than 30 mL), but it may be difficult to detect a bulge with a large or tense effusion, because in this situation, the fluid cannot be milked out of one compartment and into the other.

*Balloon test or cross-fluctuance test.* The examiner places one hand over the suprapatellar pouch and the thumb and fingers of the other hand on the medial and lateral sides of the joint line, just distal to the margins of the patella. By pressing down with one hand and then the other, the examiner may feel cross-fluctuance of the fluid under the hands (Figure 6-18). The balloon test is particularly useful for patients in whom the patellar tap (Figure 6-19) is difficult

to perform due to a large, tense effusion or the presence of a fixed knee-flexion deformity.

## Is There Pathology Involving Soft Tissues?

Palpation of muscles and tendons is helpful in determining whether the structure is inflamed or partially or completely torn, and it helps to determine atrophy, especially if one side is asymmetric compared to the opposite side. Soliciting active contraction and passively stretching the painful muscle or tendon is required to complete the evaluation.

*Quadriceps muscle and tendon.* Disuse atrophy of the **quadriceps muscle,** especially the vastus medialis component, is a common finding in patients with knee pathology. The vastus medialis is palpated for its bulk and firmness bilaterally, with the knee in extension, during voluntary contraction of the muscle. Normally, the underlying femur bone cannot be palpated through the vastus medialis muscle without the application of extraordinary pressure. The girth of the quadriceps is measured and compared bilaterally by tape measure at a defined distance (approximately 15 cm above the tibial tubercle) with the knee in extension and the muscle contracted (Figure 6-20). The vastus medialis obliquus (VMO) contributes to both medial stability of the patella

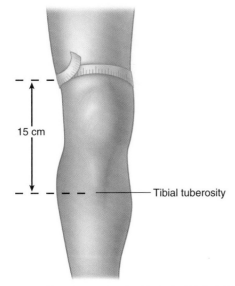

**FIGURE 6-20    MEASURING QUADRICEPS MUSCLE BULK.**

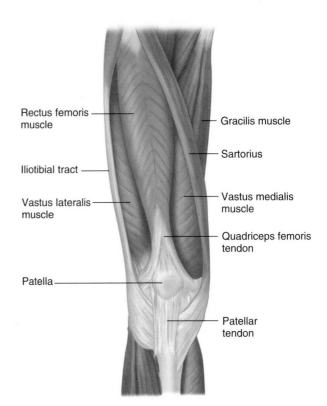

**FIGURE 6-21    QUADRICEPS TENDON.**

and the screw-home movement of the tibia on the femur in the last 10° of extension.

The **quadriceps tendon** is palpated for tenderness, defects, or swelling along the central tendinous portion and over the insertion into the proximal patellar pole. The medial and lateral patellar insertions of the vastus medialis and vastus lateralis, respectively, in association with the patellar retinacula, should also be palpated if pathology in the extensor mechanism is being considered (Figure 6-21).

*Infrapatellar ligament (patellar tendon).* Because this structure connects two bones, it is sometimes referred to as the **infrapatellar ligament.** Others consider the patella to be a large sesamoid bone and therefore refer to the structure as the **patellar tendon.** The infrapatellar ligament is palpated for tenderness, swelling, or defects along its length, from the inferior pole of the patella to its insertion into the tibial tubercle. The **infrapatellar fat pad** is situated immediately posterior to the patellar tendon at the level of the joint line. It can be readily palpated by curling the fingers around the tendon from either side (see Figure 6-8).

*Pes anserinus.* The pes anserinus—the conjoint tendon of the sartorius, gracilis, and semitendinosus muscles—inserts into the medial surface of the proximal tibia about 5 cm below the joint line and at the same level as the tibial tuberosity (see Figure 6-8). It is best palpated during resisted knee flexion of less than 90° (Figure 6-22). The fingers are placed around the medial aspect of the knee, just above the joint line. The two sharp, cordlike structures are the gracilis (more anterior and lateral) and the semitendinosus (more posterior and medial). Between these two structures, the bulky semimembranosus tendon (not part of the pes anserinus) can be palpated. More proximally, the semimembranosus muscle bulk is evident medial to the semitendinosus tendon. The fleshy bulk anterior to the gracilis tendon is the sartorius muscle.

*Iliotibial tract.* The iliotibial tract is attached proximally to the iliac crest. The tensor fascia lata muscle inserts into it anteriorly, and the bulk of the gluteus maximus muscle inserts into it posteriorly (Figure 6-23). Distally, the iliotibial band attaches to the Gerdy tubercle on the anterolateral aspect of the proximal tibia. A band from the iliotibial tract also attaches to the lateral upper patella (superior patellar retinaculum). It is easy to palpate the iliotibial band distally by moving the fingers from the posterior to anterior aspect, just anterior to the biceps femoris tendon, while the knee is flexed 30° with an ipsilateral single-leg stance or during resisted abduction of the hip (see Figure 6-23).

### Is the Iliotibial Band Inflamed?

A tight iliotibial band can be associated with iliotibial band syndrome, inflammation of the band as it crosses over the lateral femoral epicondyle. This can be assessed with the **Ober test** (described in Chapter 5) and by one of the following two tests.

*Renne test.* The iliotibial band is directly over the lateral femoral epicondyle when the knee is in approximately 30° of flexion. The patient stands with the knee extended, and the examiner's fingers are placed over the lateral femoral epicondyle. The patient is then asked to slowly flex the knee down into a squatting position (Figure 6-24). Pain at the epicondyle at about 30° of knee flexion is suggestive of **iliotibial band friction syndrome.**

*Noble test.* This test is analogous to the Renne test but with the patient supine on the examining table. The knee is passively flexed and extended with one hand around the ankle and the thumb of the other hand placed over the lateral femoral epicondyle. Pain over the epicondyle at about 30° of knee flexion is suggestive of **iliotibial band friction syndrome.**

*Semimembranosus.* The biceps femoris, the semimembranosus, and the semitendinosus together make up the hamstring muscles. The semimembranosus muscle can be palpated between the gracilis and semitendinosus tendons

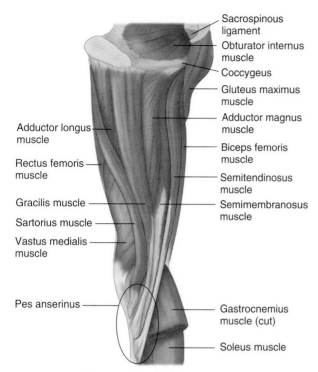

Sacrospinous ligament
Obturator internus muscle
Coccygeus
Gluteus maximus muscle
Adductor magnus muscle
Biceps femoris muscle
Semitendinosus muscle
Semimembranosus muscle

Adductor longus muscle
Rectus femoris muscle
Gracilis muscle
Sartorius muscle
Vastus medialis muscle

Pes anserinus
Gastrocnemius muscle (cut)
Soleus muscle

**FIGURE 6-22    THE ILIOTIBIAL BAND.**

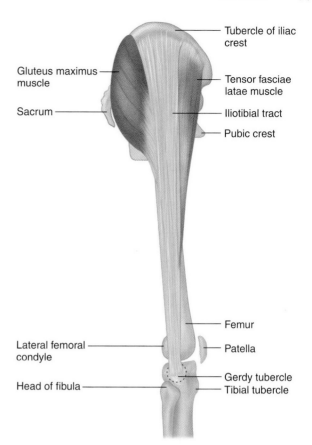

Tubercle of iliac crest
Gluteus maximus muscle
Tensor fasciae latae muscle
Sacrum
Iliotibial tract
Pubic crest

Femur
Lateral femoral condyle
Patella
Head of fibula
Gerdy tubercle
Tibial tubercle

**FIGURE 6-23    THE ILIOTIBIAL BAND.**

during resisted knee flexion in the supine or prone position. The bulky part of the muscle is medial to the semitendinosus proximally, but distally the tendon comes to lie deep to the pes anserinus as the tendon inserts more proximally onto the posteromedial tibial plateau (see Figure 6-22). It can be difficult to distinguish between semimembranosus tendinitis and posteromedial joint-line tenderness caused by meniscus pathology.

*Biceps femoris.* The biceps femoris tendon can be readily palpated in the supine or prone position, with the knee flexed, by curling the fingers around the proximal fibula and then moving them proximally around the cordlike biceps femoris tendon, which attaches to the fibular head. Resisted knee flexion makes the tendon more prominent. The common peroneal nerve can be palpated just below the biceps femoris tendon insertion, as it winds around the fibular head. The nerve is quite superficial at this level, and the patient may experience some discomfort with palpation.

*Gastrocnemius.* With the patient in the prone position and the knee flexed against resistance, the insertions of the gastrocnemius into the back of the medial and lateral femoral condyles may be palpated. Tendinitis may develop at either insertion point. The muscle belly is readily palpable more distally. The medial head of the gastrocnemius is torn more commonly than the lateral head during sports.

*Knee bursae.* A bursa is a potential space with very little fluid that facilitates movement of adjacent soft tissues. It is usually not palpable unless bursitis with fluid distension has developed. Bursae are compressible but may be quite firm to palpation. Chronic bursitis may lead to loculation of the bursa, making it difficult to aspirate. There are at least 14 bursae about the knee joint, but some are more commonly associated with clinical problems. For example, a **popliteal cyst** (Baker cyst) is readily visible and palpable with the patient standing. It is located between the medial

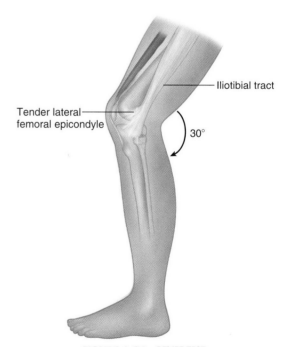

Iliotibial tract
Tender lateral femoral epicondyle
30°

**FIGURE 6-24    RENEE TEST.**

gastrocnemius insertion and the semimembranosus tendon. This cyst typically arises due to chronic knee-joint inflammation with persistent joint fluid that enters into and distends the **semimembranosus bursae.** The popliteal cyst usually maintains a connection with the knee joint, which is why aspiration usually results in recurrence unless the underlying joint pathology is also addressed. The **prepatellar bursa** lies between the patella and the overlying skin. The **deep infrapatellar bursa,** which lies distal to the infrapatellar fat pad, separates the patellar tendon from the proximal tibia. The **superficial infrapatellar bursa** is situated more superficially, between the patellar tendon and the overlying skin. Medially the **pes anserine bursa** separates the tendons of the sartorius, gracilis, and semitendinosus from the underlying tibia.

*Synovial membrane.* The synovial membrane can be palpated for tenderness and synovial swelling (thickening) in a similar fashion. The thumbs of both hands palpate the medial and lateral joint lines, with the fingers placed behind the knee for counterpressure (see Figure 6-16).

*Infrapatellar fat pad.* The infrapatellar fat pad lies immediately behind the patellar ligament at the level of the joint line. Contusion of the pad is associated with local pain, tenderness, and swelling.

### Is There Pathology Involving Bony Structures?

*Patellar pathology and tests.* The patella is readily palpable in the supine patient. The main body may be tender to palpation with traumatic contusions or fractures. Occasionally there is a **bipartite patella,** with a groove between the superolateral portion and the main patellar fragment (Figure 6-25). This can be a variant of normal. If it is associated with tenderness to palpation, swelling, or crepitus, a patellar fracture must be ruled out. Unless the patient has ligamentous laxity, the undersurface of the patella is difficult to palpate. The lateral facet can best be palpated for **retropatellar tenderness** or defects by sliding the patella laterally with the knee relaxed and extended. The medial surface can

be palpated if the patella can be flipped up to face the examiner medially. The margins of the trochlear groove of the femur can be palpated with the knee flexed and the patella displaced to either side.

The patella is subject to lateral displacement during flexion and extension because the femur meets the tibia at an angle (see Figure 6-2). Because the quadriceps pulls along the femur, and the patellar tendon is anchored along the proximal tibia, this angle tends to force the patella laterally during active extension with muscle contraction. The vastus medialis resists this lateral translation, and the distal femoral anatomic groove further prevents patellar displacement. Normally the distance between the tibial tubercle and the lower pole of the patella is approximately the same distance as the distance from the lower to the upper pole of the patella (the patellar length). A high riding patella (**patella alta**) is one in which the length from the tendon to the lower patellar pole is greater than the patellar height, causing the patella to lie above the deep part of the femoral groove. In this position the patella is more prone to lateral displacement. **Patella baja** denotes a low-lying patella. The Q angle represents the relationship between the quadriceps muscle line of pull through the patella onto the tibial tubercle. As noted previously, a large Q angle has significant implications for patellar stability and may be associated with a patellofemoral syndrome (pain in the anterior aspect of the knee related to the extensor mechanism). The combination of generalized ligamentous laxity, a large Q angle, and a high-riding patella places the individual at high risk for the development of patellofemoral syndrome.

**Chondromalacia patellae** is a pathological diagnosis of cartilage damage or softening. It may be associated with the clinical entity of patellofemoral syndrome, but the two terms are not synonymous. The line of quadriceps muscle pull is approximated by drawing a line from the anterior superior iliac spine (see Chapter 5) to the center of the patella in a supine patient with the hips and knees fully extended. The angle between this line and a line from the center of the patella to the tibial tubercle constitutes the Q angle (see Figure 6-4).

### Patellar Tests

*Patellar apprehension (instability) test.* Because of the Q angle, patellar dislocation is almost always to the lateral side. Spontaneous reduction is common before the patient presents to the examiner. With the patient in the supine position and the knee in a comfortable position of a few degrees of flexion, the patella is gently pushed laterally from its medial border. Patient apprehension and pain are evidence of previous patellar dislocation and are often accompanied by quadriceps muscle contraction. A modification of this test, known as the **moving patellar apprehension test (MPAT),** is associated with greater diagnostic accuracy. It is performed with the knee in full extension and the patella displaced laterally as far as possible by the examiner's thumb. The knee is then flexed to 90° and brought back into full extension with the lateral force maintained. The test is then repeated, but with force directed *medially.* For the MPAT to be considered positive, the patient must display apprehension with a laterally directed force but *not* with a medially directed force.

*Patellofemoral grinding test (Clarke sign).* With the patient supine, the knee extended, and the leg relaxed,

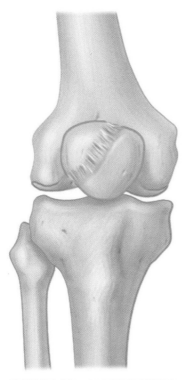

**FIGURE 6-25  A BIPARTITE PATELLA.**

the patella is pushed distally in the trochlear groove by the examiner. The patient is then asked to tighten the quadriceps while the examiner palpates, compresses, and resists proximal movement of the patella. Normally, patellar movements are smooth and painless; but in patients with patellofemoral osteoarthritis or patellar contusion, the movements are rough and painful. The maneuver can be very painful, even in normal subjects. The patellar grinding test is neither sensitive nor specific and adds little useful information.

### Is There a Pathological Plica Causing Anterior Knee Pain?

A **synovial plica** is a band of synovial tissue that is present in most normal knees. With repeated trauma or irritation, these plicae can become thickened and painful (**pathological plica**). A pathological plica often manifests as anterior knee pain that may be associated with popping or snapping sensations and may need to be considered in the differential diagnosis of anterior knee pain. A pathological plica is more common on the medial side. Rarely, a thick cord and popping of the plical band can be palpated medially by internally rotating the tibia while flexing and extending the knee joint (**Hughston plica test**). The patient may also experience apprehension as the patella is pushed medially in the supine position with the knee flexed to approximately 30°. The apprehension is caused by pain that occurs as the plica is compressed between the patella and the underlying medial femoral condyle.

*Tibial tuberosity.* The tibial tubercle is readily palpable at the inferior attachment of the patellar ligament, a few centimeters below the joint line. It may be quite prominent in individuals with a history of tibial tubercle apophysitis (Osgood-Schlatter disease).

*Medial femoral condyle and epicondyle.* The medial femoral condyle can be palpated in the flexed knee medial to the patellar ligament, from the joint line distally to the proximal extent of the condyle medial to the patella. Full knee flexion is required to palpate the inferior part of the condyle. The proximal part can best be palpated with the knee in extension and the patella displaced laterally. The medial femoral epicondyle is readily palpable a few centimeters above the joint, the most prominent medial bony landmark of the distal femur, where the MCL attaches proximally (see Figure 6-5).

*Lateral femoral condyle and epicondyle.* The lateral femoral condyle is less prominent than the medial condyle but can be palpated in an analogous manner. The lateral epicondyle is easily identified as the most prominent lateral bony landmark on the distal femur, where the fibular collateral ligament is attached proximally (see Figure 6-5). Either epicondyle may be tender if it is inflamed (epicondylitis). Inflammation of the iliotibial band may cause tenderness in this area, which can be differentiated from epicondylitis using Ober, Renne, and Noble tests as described earlier.

*Medial tibial plateau.* Beginning from the joint line adjacent to the medial side of the patellar ligament, the fingers are moved medially to palpate the prominent medial tibial plateau (see Figure 6-16). The posterior muscular attachments prevent bony palpation of the posteromedial plateau in most patients. Osteoarthritis may lead to osteophyte formation around the knee joint, which may be readily palpable as enlargements that may or may not be tender.

*Lateral tibial plateau.* The joint line and plateau are palpated beginning at the lateral margin of the patellar ligament and moving laterally along the lateral tibial plateau (see Figure 6-16). As on the posteromedial side, the posterolateral plateau is difficult to palpate because of the muscular and tendinous structures overlying it.

*Lateral tibial (Gerdy) tubercle.* The iliotibial tract inserts into the Gerdy tubercle just below the joint line, between the fibular head laterally and the patellar ligament medially (see Figure 6-1). It is quite distinct in some individuals.

*Fibular head.* The fibular head is readily palpated by following the biceps femoris tendon distally, from behind the lateral aspect of the femur to its insertion into the fibular head. The fibular head becomes more distinct with internal rotation of the tibia on the femur. The fibular head may be grasped between the thumb and fingers to test for stability and inflammation of the proximal tibiofibular joint by attempting to displace the fibula forward and backward. The common peroneal nerve can be palpated by moving the fingers distally along the proximal fibula until a cordlike structure is noted crossing the bone obliquely. The nerve can be rolled and palpated gently with the fingers; firm palpation may cause pain and paresthesia.

### Is There Joint Instability or Pathology Involving the Ligaments?

The medial and lateral collateral ligaments are the main structures that resist varus and valgus forces across the knee joint, whereas the anterior cruciate ligament resists primarily anterior translation of the tibia relative to the femur, and the posterior cruciate ligament primarily resists posterior translation of the tibia relative to the femur. The collateral ligaments can be assessed by palpation and other maneuvers, but the cruciate ligaments cannot be directly palpated and are evaluated indirectly through various specific maneuvers.

### Medial and Lateral Collateral Ligament Palpation

When palpating the MCL, it may be difficult to differentiate meniscal tenderness in the medial joint line from MCL tenderness, given the intimate relationship between these two structures (see Figures 6-6 and 6-9). It is important to assess the entire extent of the ligament by slowly moving from the medial femoral epicondyle down to the tibial insertion point. The area of maximal tenderness should be sought. Maximal tenderness over the ligament, away from the joint line, is less likely to be related to meniscus pathology.

The LCL is easily isolated by placing the leg into the figure-four position. The ligament can then be palpated as it runs from the lateral femoral epicondyle to the fibular head. It is situated anterior to the biceps femoris tendon distally (Figure 6-26).

### Joint Stability

In most slightly flexed, normal knees, some laxity allows a few degrees of angulation in varus/valgus testing and a few millimeters of **glide** in the anteroposterior plane. When examining a patient with an acute injury, laxity may be difficult to detect due to muscle spasm. The patient should be made as comfortable as possible to facilitate muscle relaxation, especially of the hamstring and quadriceps muscles.

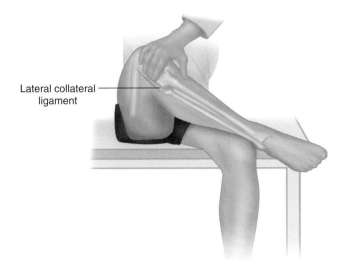

Lateral collateral
ligament

**FIGURE 6-26    PALPATION OF LATERAL COLLATERAL LIGAMENT.**

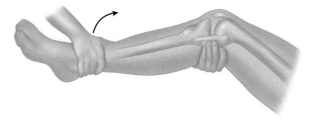

**FIGURE 6-27    TESTING MCL.**

*Severity of ligament injury.* Ligament injuries are graded from first degree to third degree. **First-degree injuries** involve microscopic tearing of the ligament that results in mild swelling and pain with palpation and stressing but no joint instability. **Second-degree injuries** involve microscopic tears of a portion of the ligament with pain on palpation and stressing of the ligament, along with moderate swelling and bruising and a slight instability of a firm end point. A **third-degree tear** is a complete tear of the ligament that involves considerable swelling and bruising with gross instability but may actually be associated with less pain on palpation and stressing of the ligament than a lesser, second-degree injury.

*Pseudolaxity and fixed deformity.* Care must be taken to consider the neutral, varus/valgus, and anterior/posterior positions of the knee in relation to the start and end positions of the ligament test. Loss of articular cartilage and collapse of a knee compartment due to arthritis may result in increased movement with varus/valgus testing, as the knee is brought from its deformed position to a normal position. This phenomenon is observed when the ligament retains its normal length in the presence of collapse of the corresponding joint compartment, known as **pseudolaxity**. If the collapse is long-standing, the corresponding ligament may contract, resulting in a **fixed deformity**. Similarly, a rupture of the PCL results in **posterior sag** of the tibia and an apparent increased anterior translation of the tibia in a forward direction. If the examiner does not appreciate that the start position is abnormal, anterior laxity may be mistakenly diagnosed.

*Medial stability.* The MCL and the posteromedial capsule provide the major static medial support to the knee joint. At 30° of flexion, the MCL is isolated, whereas the posteromedial capsule and cruciate ligaments contribute to the resistance of valgus force in full-knee extension. The medial joint line is palpated while the leg is supported. With the knee at 30° of flexion, a valgus force is applied by the examiner's arms (Figure 6-27). Joint opening and the patient's pain response during valgus stressing of the joint are noted. Repeating the test with the knee in full extension evaluates both the MCL and the posterior capsule. If there is laxity in both flexion and full extension, both structures, and possibly one or more cruciate ligaments, are torn. If there is laxity only at 30° of flexion, the posterior capsule is intact.

*Lateral stability.* The LCL and the posterolateral knee-joint capsule provide the major static resistance to varus forces at the knee joint. Isolated injury to the LCL is rare, and associated tests for the posterior capsular structures (see Posterolateral Instability, p. 86) should always be performed when considering lateral-sided knee instability. The capsule and the cruciate ligaments provide strong resistance to varus force in knee extension, whereas the LCL acts more in isolation with knee flexion. To isolate the LCL, the knee is flexed to 30°, the lateral joint line is palpated, and a varus force is applied using the leg tucked under the examiner's arm as a fulcrum. The tibia should be kept in neutral rotation. The test is repeated in full-knee extension to evaluate the integrity of the posterior capsule. Laxity in both flexion and extension suggests disruption of the posterior capsule, and possibly of one or more cruciate ligaments, along with the LCL. The patient's pain response is assessed during ligament stress testing. A grade 1 ligament tear will exhibit no laxity, but the patient will experience pain with stressing.

*Anterior stability.* The ACL prevents forward displacement of the tibia on the femur. It is taut with internal tibial rotation. This structure may be injured during running, when the foot is planted and the individual pivots to the same side, resulting in strong internal tibial rotation on the femur. The ACL may also be injured with hyperextension, as the tibia is forced forward on the femur, or with a direct blow to the tibia from behind.

*Lachman test.* After an acute injury, hamstring spasm will prevent the examiner from appreciating laxity of the ACL with the knee in flexion. Moreover, it may be difficult for the patient to flex the knee due to pain. A Lachman test can be performed supine or prone with the knee in a comfortable position of slight flexion (about 30°). The femur is stabilized with one hand, while the other is used to pull the proximal tibia forward. It is important for the patient to try to relax the hamstring muscles during this test, but it is less critical; the hamstrings are at a mechanical disadvantage, because the examiner's force is being applied roughly perpendicular to the muscle line of pull (Figure 6-28).

*Anterior drawer test.* The anterior drawer test is performed with the knee flexed 90° and the hip flexed 45°. The **passive anterior drawer test** involves placing the examiner's fingers up the proximal tibia and fibula into the hamstrings, to make sure that these are relaxed. An anterior force is then applied to the proximal tibia, in an attempt to displace it forward on the femur, while the foot is stabilized on the examination table (Figure 6-29). Hamstring spasm can yield

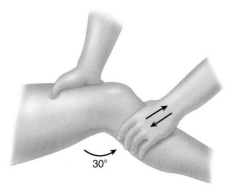

**FIGURE 6-28   LACHMAN TEST.**

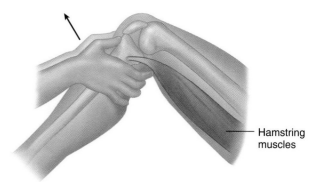

**FIGURE 6-29   ANTERIOR DRAWER TEST.**

Hamstring muscles

a false-negative result. The **active anterior drawer test** can be performed with the knee in the same position. It involves stabilizing the foot and asking the patient to contract the quadriceps to try to extend the leg against resistance. The quadriceps muscles pull the tibia forward if the ACL is disrupted. The active anterior drawer test is unlikely to yield useful information in an acutely painful injury because of quadriceps inhibition due to pain.

### Anteromedial and Anterolateral Rotatory Instability

*Pivot shift (MacIntosh) test and jerk test of Hughston.* The **pivot shift test (MacIntosh test)** is a test for anterolateral rotatory instability caused by **both an anterior cruciate tear and a posterolateral capsular tear.** With the knee in full extension, the tibia internally rotated, and a valgus force applied, the tibia and the fibular head will sublux forward on the femur laterally in the presence of a complete ACL tear combined with a posterolateral capsule tear. As the knee joint is flexed beyond 30° to 40°, the iliotibial band comes to lie posterior to the lateral femoral epicondyle, and the tibia is seen to jump backward into position due to traction from the iliotibial band and other secondary restraints pulling the tibia back into place (Figure 6-30). The degree of instability is increased with hip abduction, because it relaxes the iliotibial tract. With severe disruption of the posterolateral corner of the knee joint, the tibia may jam up against the femoral condyle and not reduce until the valgus stress is relaxed, allowing further knee flexion. In the presence of medial joint instability, the pivot shift test cannot be performed, because the essential medial fulcrum is lost. After the tibia is reduced with flexion, the examiner can extend the knee again, while maintaining the valgus and internal rotation force at the knee. The tibia is seen and felt to jerk anteriorly, as it displaces once more at about 30°. This maneuver is sometimes called the **jerk test of Hughston.** It is less sensitive than the pivot shift test.

*Slocum test.* **ACL disruptions** are commonly associated with anterior rotatory instability because of disruption of both the ACL and the posteromedial capsule (**anteromedial rotatory instability**) or the posterolateral capsule (**anterolateral rotatory instability**). Testing for posterior capsular injury with the Slocum test involves performing the anterior drawer test with the hip flexed 45° and the knee flexed 90° with the tibia either in external rotation, to tighten the posteromedial capsule, or in internal rotation, to evaluate the integrity of the posterolateral capsule (Figure 6-31). The

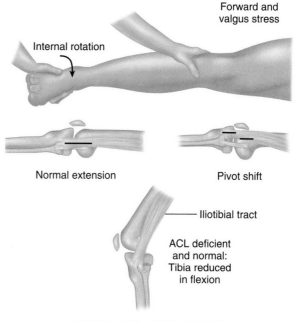

Forward and valgus stress

Internal rotation

Normal extension        Pivot shift

Iliotibial tract

ACL deficient and normal: Tibia reduced in flexion

**FIGURE 6-30   PIVOT SHIFT TEST.**

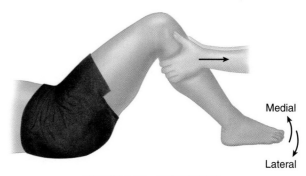

Medial

Lateral

**FIGURE 6-31   SLOCUM TEST.**

tibia should be rotated no more than 15° to 20° to avoid excessive tightening of multiple secondary restraints that might lead to a false-negative test. If the capsule is intact, the drawer should be *greater* in the neutral position than when the capsule is tightened in internal or external rotation. Anterolateral rotatory instability exists if the amount of anterior laxity in internal rotation is similar to that of the anterior drawer test done in the neutral position. Anteromedial rotatory instability exists if the amount of anterior laxity

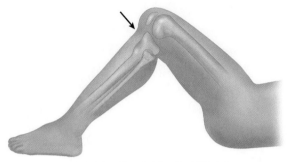

FIGURE 6-32    POSTERIOR SAG TEST.

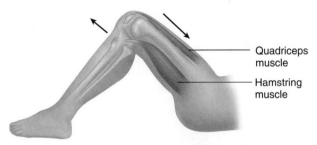

FIGURE 6-33    QUADRICEPS ACTIVE TEST.

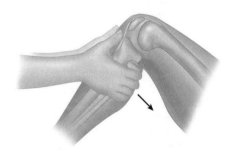

FIGURE 6-34    POSTERIOR DRAWER TEST.

in external rotation is similar to that of the anterior drawer test done in the neutral position (see Figure 6-31).

## Posterior Stability

The PCL prevents posterior displacement of the tibia on the femur; however, the PCL can be disrupted during sports, when an individual falls onto a hyperflexed knee, or when the tibia is forced posteriorly while the leg is planted. The latter mechanism may also occur during a motor vehicle collision, as the engine and dash impact against the proximal tibia, forcing it posteriorly relative to the femur. The PCL may also be injured with the knee in hyperextension, although this mechanism usually results in combined injuries. Knee hyperextension first disrupts the ACL, followed by the posterior capsule and ultimately the PCL.

It is important to remember that examination of the patient in the supine position subjects the PCL-deficient knee to the forces of gravity, with the result that the tibia may be in the displaced position when the knee is first evaluated. It is not uncommon for junior clinicians to mistakenly diagnose ACL deficiency in a PCL-deficient knee.

*Posterior sag (gravity drawer test) and quadriceps active test.* Normally, the tibial plateau is visible and palpable in front of the medial and lateral femoral condyles with the knee in 90° of flexion. With the patient supine, the hip flexed 45°, and the knee flexed 90°, the tibia will sag backward due to gravity if the PCL is incompetent (Figure 6-32). When looking for posterior sag, care should be taken to position the tibia in neutral rotation to avoid involving the secondary restraints of the knee, which could lead to a false-negative test. The examiner can look for a **posterior sag** of the tibia by lifting the patient's heel until the hip and knee are in 90° of flexion, taking into consideration the neutral position of the tibia in relation to the femur. A sagging tibia can be lifted forward to the neutral position. Alternatively, the patient may be asked to contract the quadriceps muscle to lift the tibia forward to the neutral position. This maneuver is sometimes referred to as the **quadriceps active test** (Figure 6-33). Care should be taken to avoid misinterpreting the anterior translation observed as a positive active anterior drawer sign (see the earlier discussion of the anterior drawer sign), which indicates disruption of the ACL. The key is to note whether the tibia begins in a posteriorly displaced position (PCL rupture with posterior sag due to gravity) or in a normal position (normal or ACL rupture) before the anterior translation is noted, and whether it lies in a normal position (PCL rupture reduced by quadriceps) or in an anteriorly displaced position (ACL rupture) when the quadriceps muscle is actively pulling the tibia forward.

*Reverse Lachman test.* The concept is the same as for the Lachman test, except that the force is directed posteriorly, beginning with the knee flexed 30° and the tibia in a neutral position. In practice, the Lachman and reverse Lachman tests are performed at the same time by alternately applying an anterior force and then a posterior force, taking care to note the neutral position of the tibia on the femur and to interpret any translation in relation to this position.

*Posterior drawer test.* The **posterior drawer test** can be performed actively and passively, as with the anterior drawer test, except that the force is directed posteriorly. Comparison is always made with the normal side. As with the anterior drawer test, the knee is flexed 90° with the tibia in neutral rotation. With the fingers palpating the tibial plateau and femoral condyles anteriorly to assess their relative position, the proximal tibia is pulled forward until the tibia is in the normal relationship to the femur (tibial plateau palpable about 1 cm in front of the femoral condyles). A posteriorly directed force is then applied to the proximal tibia, and the degree of posterior translation is noted. Translation of the tibial plateau to a position posterior to the femoral condyles indicates complete disruption of the PCL (Figure 6-34). In practice, the anterior and posterior drawer tests are usually performed at the same time.

The **active posterior drawer test** can be performed with the knee in the same position. The foot is stabilized on the examination table, and the patient attempts to flex the knee. The hamstrings will pull the tibia posteriorly into a maximally displaced position in a PCL-deficient knee. The examiner must recognize that the tibia usually starts from a displaced position already, due to gravity. A positive result will be more evident if the tibia is passively reduced to a neutral position before hamstring contraction.

## Posteromedial and Posterolateral Rotatory Instability

**PCL disruptions** are commonly associated with posterior rotatory instability because of concomitant disruption of the posteromedial capsule (**posteromedial rotatory instability**) or, more commonly, the posterolateral capsule (**posterolateral rotatory instability**). Although these rotatory tests are analogous to those discussed earlier for anterior rotatory instability, the junior clinician may be confused by the fact that the opposite tibial rotation is required to test the posterolateral (or posteromedial) corner. Consideration of the force to be applied will remind the examiner of the correct rotation for each test: If *anterior stability* is to be tested, by applying an anteriorly directed force, external rotation of the tibia will slacken the posterolateral structures and tighten up the posteromedial structures. If *posterior stability* is to be tested, by applying a posteriorly directed force, external tibial rotation will tighten up the posterolateral structures and slacken the posteromedial ones once the force is applied.

Testing for **posterior capsular injury** involves performing the posterior drawer test with the tibia either in external rotation, to tighten the posterolateral capsule, or in internal rotation, to evaluate the integrity of the posteromedial capsule. The tibia should be rotated no more than 15° to 20° to avoid excessive tightening of multiple secondary restraints, which might lead to a false-negative test. If the capsule is intact, the drawer should be *greater* in the neutral position than when the capsule is tightened in internal or external rotation. Posterolateral rotatory instability exists if the amount of posterior laxity in external rotation is similar to that of the posterior drawer test done in the neutral position. Posteromedial rotatory instability exists if the amount of posterior laxity in internal rotation is similar to that of the posterior drawer test done in the neutral position.

*Reverse pivot shift test.* This is a test of posterolateral rotatory instability; it follows the same concept as the pivot shift test but for the PCL. With the knee flexed 70° to 80° and the patient in the supine position, an external rotation and valgus force are applied to the tibia. This forces the tibia into a subluxed position if the PCL and posterolateral corner of the knee are disrupted. While the valgus and external tibial rotation are maintained, the knee is extended. Visible and palpable reduction of the tibia occurs as the knee nears full extension. The test can also be performed with the patient in the prone position, and it can be performed with the knee reduced in full extension; the subluxation is observed as the knee is flexed upward, analogous to the jerk test.

*Tibial external rotation (dial) test.* Disruption of the posterolateral corner of the knee results in excessive external tibial rotation. With the patient in the prone position, and the knees in 30° of flexion, both feet are passively externally rotated by lifting the great toes (Figure 6-35). More than 10° of excess external rotation indicates the presence of a torn posterolateral knee capsule and surrounding structures. The test should then be repeated with 90° of knee flexion. An isolated posterolateral capsular injury is associated with less side-to-side difference in rotation at 90°, because the intact PCL provides stability in 90° of knee flexion. If the posterolateral capsular injury is associated with a PCL disruption, the test will be equally or more positive with the knee flexed 90°, compared with 30° of flexion. A negative test in 30° of flexion implies that no significant injury is present to the posterolateral corner, and the 90° test is not required.

*External rotation recurvatum test.* With the patient in the supine position, the legs are lifted off the examining table by the great toes. The amount of external tibial rotation and knee recurvatum are noted. Excessive lateral rotation

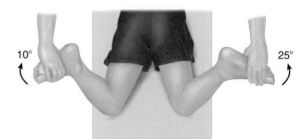

**FIGURE 6-35  TIBIAL EXTERNAL (DIAL) TEST.**

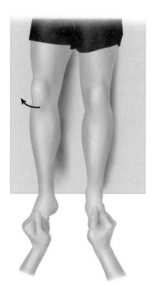

**FIGURE 6-36  EXTERNAL ROTATION RECURVATUM TEST.**

is indicative of a **posterolateral capsular injury**. Excessive rotation combined with recurvatum suggests a combined injury to the posterolateral corner of the knee and one or more of the cruciate ligaments. The examiner should be aware that external rotation may give the appearance of genu varum (Figure 6-36).

### Is There Pathology Involving the Menisci?

The menisci are situated between the femur and tibia, allowing the outer edge to be palpated along the medial and lateral joint line. Joint-line tenderness alone is not very specific, as it may be related to other problems, such as arthritic involvement of the medial or lateral compartment. Several specific maneuvers have been described that aim to detect meniscus pathology.

### Medial and Lateral Meniscus Palpation

Palpation along the medial and lateral joint lines is performed with the patient in the supine or sitting position with the knee flexed 90° and the muscles relaxed. Palpation proceeds from the patellar ligament anteriorly to the biceps femoris tendon laterally and the semitendinosus medially. The posterior horn of the meniscus is easier to palpate with the patient prone. The posterior horn of the lateral meniscus is palpated posteromedial to the biceps femoris tendon, and the posterior horn of the medial meniscus can be palpated posterolateral to the semimembranosus tendon.

### Meniscal Tests

*McMurray test.* The basic premise of the McMurray test is that meniscus tears are trapped during certain knee movements, with resultant pain and clunking. The test is easy to demonstrate but difficult to describe. It can be properly performed only if the patient has a reasonably full and relatively pain-free range of motion. The knee is flexed to 90°, and an external rotation and varus force are applied to the joint. The applied forces are maintained while the knee is flexed smoothly to a position of maximum flexion, and then the force is smoothly changed from a varus and external rotation force to an internal rotation and valgus force while the knee is extended from the fully flexed position. The process is then reversed and is usually repeated several times in smooth succession, until the examiner is satisfied that the entire range has been thoroughly assessed. It may be helpful to consider that the heel describes a large "U," with the toes always pointing toward the center of the "U." During the test, the fingers of the examiner's free hand are placed along the medial and lateral joint lines to palpate any abnormal snapping or clicking that might be caused by meniscus pathology. A positive test is indicated by pain in association with a clunk, as the torn meniscus fragment is manipulated between the femur and tibia. It is possible to trap a meniscus fragment and cause the knee to lock completely. Although it is generally thought that the medial meniscus is assessed during the valgus and internal rotation position of the tibia, and the lateral meniscus during the opposite phase of the test, this is probably an oversimplification. The area of pain and clunking is more reliable in pointing out the location of pathology in conjunction with other signs and symptoms (Figure 6-37).

*Apley distraction and grinding (compression) tests.* Joint-line tenderness can be associated with meniscus or collateral ligament injury. The concept behind the Apley test is that ligaments usually are painful when stressed in distraction, whereas pain involving the meniscus is felt with compression. With the patient in the prone position, the knee flexed 90°, and the femur stabilized with one hand, distraction is applied with the other hand by pulling upward on the ankle while rotating medially and laterally. A varus and valgus force may also be applied to further delineate whether the MCL or the LCL might be the source of pain (**Apley distraction test**). Once the distraction portion of the test has been completed, compression is applied to alternately grind the medial and lateral meniscus between the tibia and femur, with gentle varus and valgus force applied, while internally and externally rotating and compressing the ankle downward (**Apley grinding or compression test**; Figure 6-38).

*Duck walk test (Childress sign).* The squatting position places great stress on the posterior horns of both menisci and is painful if the posterior horn is torn. The patient is asked to squat and "walk like a duck." Pain in combination with a clunk suggests a posterior horn meniscus tear.

### KNEE RANGE OF MOVEMENT

### Flexion, Extension, and Rotation

Besides flexion and extension, the normal knee joint allows for internal and external rotation of the tibia on the femur, especially during knee flexion. Active and passive range-of-motion testing can be quickly screened by asking the

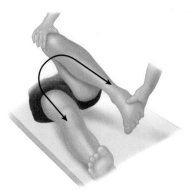

**FIGURE 6-37 McMURRAY TEST.**

patient to fully flex the knee and then extend it. The limits of motion are probed with further passive maneuvers after the maximal active range is established. Flexion and extension can be evaluated with the patient supine, prone, or standing, by asking the patient to squat. Any loss of full extension is abnormal. The range of flexion is somewhat variable, and the two sides should be compared. Lack of active full extension that can be corrected passively is usually caused by quadriceps weakness, loss of mechanical advantage, adhesion formation, effusion, or reflex inhibition. This is referred to as **extension or quadriceps lag.** Passive knee extension requires that the femur be stabilized on the examining table in the supine position, while the examiner attempts to lift the heel off the table. Although an extension lag can be passively corrected, it is not possible to correct a fixed knee-flexion deformity. Up to 5° of hyperextension at the knee is not uncommon. More than 10° of hyperextension is abnormal and suggests a cruciate ligament injury or a connective tissue disorder. Most patients are able to flex to the point of touching the heel to the buttock (approximately 135°).

**Tibial rotation** on the femur is best tested with the patient in the sitting position and the lower leg over the edge of the examining table. The patient is asked to internally rotate the lower leg and then to externally rotate it. Normally, approximately 30° internal rotation and 20° external rotation are possible. Passive manipulation is again used after the limit of active range has been observed (Figure 6-39). Normally, in full extension the tibia externally rotates on the femur into a stable position (the screw-home mechanism).

With the knee flexed 90°, any tibial torsion is noted. Normally, the forefoot points straight forward. With **medial tibial torsion,** the feet point toward each other ("pigeon-toed" foot deformity); this is often associated with genu varum. In excessive **lateral tibial torsion,** the feet point outward, and there is often a valgus deformity.

## Knee Aspiration and Joint Injection

### ARTHROCENTESIS OF THE KNEE JOINT

As a subcutaneous joint, the knee is relatively easy to aspirate through a medial retropatellar, lateral retropatellar, suprapatellar, or anterior approach. With the knee in extension, fluid accumulates in the suprapatellar pouch, where it can be aspirated. The knee should be placed into a comfortable

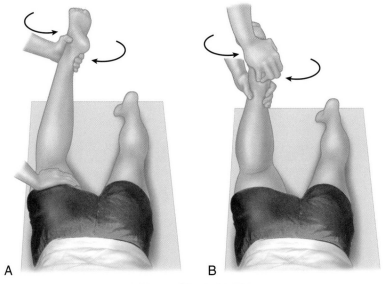

**FIGURE 6-38  APLEY TEST.**

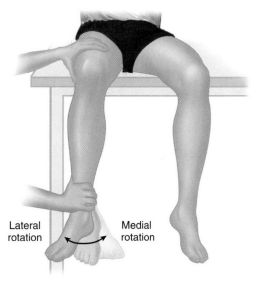

**FIGURE 6-39  PASSIVE LATERAL AND MEDIAL ROTATION OF THE KNEE.**

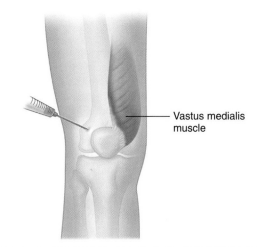

Vastus medialis muscle

**FIGURE 6-40  INJECTION OF THE KNEE: LATERAL RETROPATELLAR APPROACH.**

position of extension before beginning. It is important that the patient be relaxed and not actively contracting the quadriceps muscle. Medially, the bulk of the medial quadriceps should be avoided, because transmuscular needle insertion is painful and can cause excessive bleeding and bruising. For the **medial retropatellar approach,** the needle is inserted below the vastus medialis bulk, between the medial femoral condyle and the midpoint of the patella. Directing the needle cephalad safely places it into the suprapatellar pouch with minimal risk of injuring the patellar or femoral cartilage. Many clinicians prefer the **lateral retropatellar approach,** because there is no muscle bulk to contend with: A 21 gauge needle is inserted laterally at the junction of the middle and upper thirds of the patella, midway between the patella and the femoral condyle. If a large effusion is present, the needle is directed medially at 90° to the femur to access the suprapatellar pouch. If there is less fluid, the needle may need to be directed inferiorly and medially to enter the patellofemoral

joint before fluid is encountered (Figure 6-40). Care should be taken to minimize trauma to the cartilage of the patella and femoral condyle by advancing the needle gently between the bone surfaces and redirecting it carefully if bone is encountered before fluid can be aspirated.

A **suprapatellar approach** is indicated if there is a very large effusion expanding the suprapatellar pouch. The needle is introduced into the suprapatellar pouch, above and just lateral to the patella. In the **anterior approach,** direct access to the medial or lateral tibiofemoral joint can be obtained with the patient in a seated position and the knee flexed 90°, preferably with the leg hanging over the end of the examining table to distract the joint by gravity as much as possible. The needle is inserted about one finger's breadth above the joint line and one finger's breadth lateral or medial to the patellar ligament. The needle is directed posteriorly and parallel to the line of the tibial plateau toward the midline, aiming for an imaginary point between the inferior aspects of the femoral condyles (Figure 6-41). The anterior approach is particularly indicated for patients with fixed knee-flexion deformity.

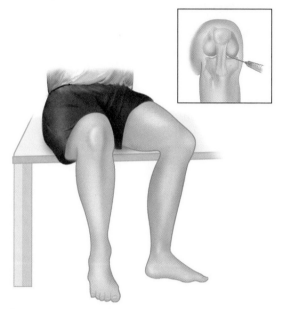

**FIGURE 6-41 INJECTION OF THE KNEE: ANTERIOR APPROACH.**

## BURSAL ASPIRATION

The prepatellar, deep infrapatellar, and anserine bursae can be aspirated and injected by placing the needle into the area of maximal fluctuance (Figure 6-42). Chronic bursitis can result in bursal loculation, which may preclude complete aspiration of fluid. The **prepatellar bursa** is injected at the center of maximal fluctuance, usually over the lower part of the patella, with the needle at a 30° angle (see Figure 6-42A). The **deep infrapatellar bursa** can be entered through a medial or lateral approach deep to the patellar ligament, proximal to its insertion into the tibial tuberosity. The **anserine bursa** is located over the anteromedial surface of the proximal tibia at the level of the tibial tuberosity. The needle is inserted into the area of maximal tenderness and fluctuance (see Figure 6-42B). A swollen popliteal bursa (cyst) is almost always caused by knee effusion with a communicating, fluid-distended medial gastrocnemius-semimembranosus bursa. Appropriate management consists of joint aspiration and treatment of the underlying knee pathology; direct aspiration or injection of a popliteal cyst is not recommended.

## ILIOTIBIAL BAND FRICTION SYNDROME

In the iliotibial band friction syndrome, the most tender site over the lateral epicondyle, where the band slips over backward and forward during knee flexion and extension, is injected (see Figure 6-42C).

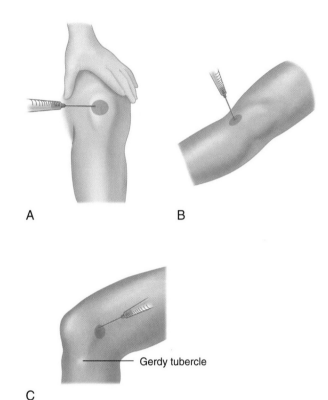

Gerdy tubercle

C

**FIGURE 6-42 INJECTIONS FOR ILIOTIBIAL BAND (ITB) FRICTION SYNDROME. A,** Prepatellar bursa. **B,** Anserine bursa. **C,** Lateral femoral epicondyle.

## SELECTED READINGS

Ahmad, C.S., McCarthy, M., Gomez, J.A., Stein, B.E.S., 2009. The moving patellar apprehension test for lateral patellar instability. Am. J. Sports Med. 37, 791–796.

Barton, T.M., Torg, J.S., Das, M., 1984. Posterior cruciate ligament insufficiency: A review of the literature. Sports Med. 16, 419–430.

Gross, J., Fetto, J., Rosen, E., 2002. Musculoskeletal Examination, second ed. Blackwell Publishing, Malden, MA.

Harris, N., 2003. Advanced Examination Techniques in Orthopaedics. Greenwich Medical Media.

Magee, D.J., 2002. Orthopedic Physical Assessment, fourth ed. WB Saunders, Philadelphia.

Malanga, G.A., Andrus, S., Nadler, S.F., McLean, J., 2003. Physical examination of the knee: A review of the original test description and scientific validity of common orthopedic tests. Arch. Phys. Med. Rehabil. 84, 592–603.

Scholten, R.J., Opstelten, W., van der Plas, C.G., et al., 2003. Accuracy of physical diagnostic tests for assessing ruptures of the anterior cruciate ligament: A meta-analysis. J. Fam. Pract. 52, 689–694.

Solomon, D.H., Simel, D.L., Bates, D.W., et al., 2001. Does this patient have a torn meniscus or ligament of the knee? Value of the physical examination. J. Am. Med. Assoc. 286, 1610–1620.

# 7

# THE ANKLE AND FOOT

David J. G. Stephen • Gregory W. Choy • Adel G. Fam

## Overview

The ankles and feet are well structured for bipedal gait. Each side must be able to independently support the entire body weight for optimal ambulation. A large number of bones, ligaments, muscles, and tendons work in concert to provide stability and flexibility through a range of activities. They include ambulating, on level or uneven ground; jumping, both lifting off and landing; kicking or striking objects with different parts of foot; and many others.

Readers should keep in mind that various systemic conditions, such as diabetes and peripheral vascular disease, have a considerable impact on the integrity of the ankle and foot. In addition, the choice of footwear, especially some designed for aesthetics rather than mechanics, can affect the function of the ankle and foot. This chapter will focus on the applied anatomy, physical examination, and common musculoskeletal (MSK) disorders of the ankle and foot.

## Applied Anatomy

The foot can be divided into three units: the *hindfoot, midfoot,* and *forefoot* (Figure 7-1). The **hindfoot** comprises the calcaneus and talus. The anterior two thirds of the calcaneus articulates with the talus, and the posterior third forms the heel. Medially, the sustentaculum tali supports the talus and is joined to the navicular bone by the **spring ligament.** The talus articulates with the tibia and fibula above at the **ankle joint,** with the calcaneus below at the **subtalar joint,** and with the navicular in front at the **talonavicular joint.**

The midfoot is made up of five tarsal bones: the *navicular* medially, the *cuboid* laterally, and the three *cuneiforms* distally. The midfoot is separated from the hindfoot by the **midtarsal or transverse tarsal joint** (talonavicular and calcaneocuboid articulations) and from the forefoot by the **tarsometatarsal joints** (see Figure 7-1).

The **forefoot** comprises the metatarsals and phalanges. The great toe has two phalanges and two sesamoids embedded in the plantar ligament under the metatarsal head. Each of the other toes has three phalanges.

The **distal tibiofibular joint** is a fibrous joint (syndesmosis) between the distal tibia and the fibula (Figure 7-2). The joint allows only slight malleolar separation (< 2 mm) on full dorsiflexion of the ankle.

### ANKLE JOINT

The **true ankle (talocrural) joint** is a saddle-shaped hinge joint between the distal ends of the tibia and fibula and the trochlea of the talus (see Figure 7-2). Most of the body weight is transmitted through the tibia to the talus. The medial (tibial) malleolus and the lateral (fibular) malleolus extend distally to form the ankle mortise that stabilizes the

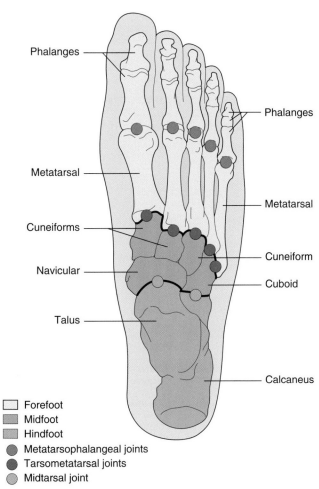

Phalanges

Phalanges

Metatarsal

Metatarsal

Cuneiforms

Cuneiform

Navicular

Cuboid

Talus

Calcaneus

☐ Forefoot
▨ Midfoot
▨ Hindfoot
● Metatarsophalangeal joints
● Tarsometatarsal joints
● Midtarsal joint

**FIGURE 7-1   THE BONES OF THE FOOT (SUPERIOR VIEW).** (From Hochberg H, Silman AJ, Smolen JS, et al., eds. *Rheumatology,* 3rd ed. Edinburgh, UK: Mosby, 2003.)

talus and prevents rotation. The joint capsule is lax anteriorly and posteriorly but is strengthened medially by the powerful **deltoid ligament** and laterally by three distinct bands: the *anterior* and *posterior talofibular ligaments* and the *calcaneofibular ligament*. The **synovial cavity** does not normally communicate with other joints, adjacent tendon sheaths, or bursae. Tendons crossing the ankle region are invested for part of their course in tenosynovial sheaths (Figures 7-3 and 7-4).

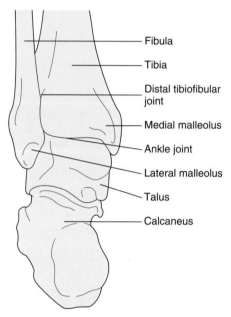

**FIGURE 7-2    THE BONES OF THE HINDFOOT (POSTERIOR VIEW).** (From Hochberg H, Silman AJ, Smolen JS, et al., eds. *Rheumatology*, 3rd ed. Edinburgh, UK: Mosby, 2003.)

In the **anterior (extensor) compartment,** the tendons of the tibialis anterior (most medial), extensor hallucis longus, extensor digitorum longus, and peroneus tertius (most lateral) muscles are bound down by the superior and inferior extensor retinaculi (see Figure 7-3). The dorsalis pedis artery runs between the extensor hallucis longus and extensor digitorum longus tendons.

In the **lateral (peroneal) compartment,** the peroneus longus and brevis tendons are enclosed in a single synovial sheath that runs behind and below the lateral malleolus (see Figure 7-3). The superior and inferior peroneal retinaculi strap down the peroneal tendons.

In the **medial (flexor) compartment,** the tendons of the tibialis posterior (most medial), flexor digitorum longus, and flexor hallucis longus (most lateral) muscles are held down by the flexor retinaculum, forming the **tarsal tunnel** (see Figure 7-4). The flexor retinaculum bridges the interval between the medial malleolus and the calcaneus. The posterior tibial artery and nerve lie between the tendons of the flexor digitorum longus and the flexor hallucis longus.

Posteriorly, the common tendon of the gastrocnemius and soleus (**Achilles tendon** or **tendocalcaneus**) is inserted into the posterior surface of the calcaneus. The tendon does not have a synovial sheath but is surrounded by a loose connective tissue known as *paratendon* or *peritenon*. The tendon of the **plantaris** muscle, which originates from the lateral femoral epicondyle and lateral meniscus, runs obliquely between the soleus and gastrocnemius muscles to insert into the medial aspect of the superior calcaneal tuberosity medial to the Achilles tendon.

Several **bursae** exist around the ankle (Figure 7-5; also see Figures 7-3 and 7-4). The retrocalcaneal bursa, located between the Achilles tendon insertion and the posterior surface of the calcaneus, is surrounded anteriorly by Kager's fat pad. The bursa serves to protect the distal Achilles

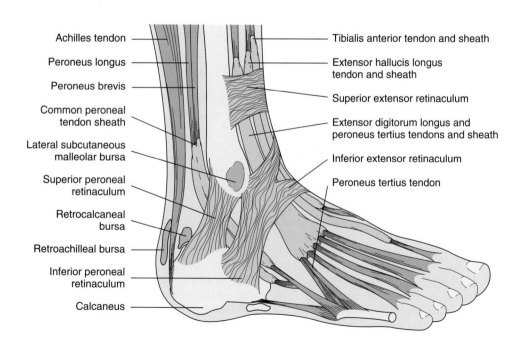

**FIGURE 7-3    BURSAE, TENDONS, AND TENDON SHEATHS OF THE ANTERIOR (EXTENSOR) AND PERONEAL COMPARTMENTS OF THE ANKLE.** (From Hochberg H, Silman AJ, Smolen JS, et al., eds. *Rheumatology*, 3rd ed. Edinburgh, UK: Mosby, 2003.)

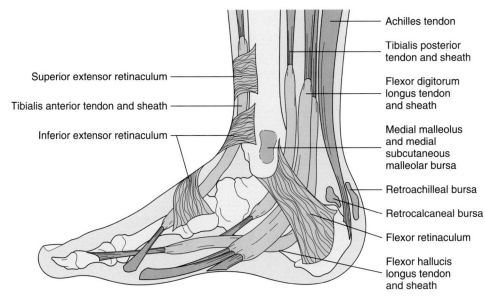

**FIGURE 7-4** **BURSAE, TENDONS, AND TENDON SHEATHS OF THE MEDIAL (FLEXOR) COMPARTMENT OF THE ANKLE.** (From Hochberg H, Silman AJ, Smolen JS, et al., eds. *Rheumatology*, 3rd ed. Edinburgh, UK: Mosby, 2003.)

*Labels in figure:*
- Achilles tendon
- Tibialis posterior tendon and sheath
- Flexor digitorum longus tendon and sheath
- Medial malleolus and medial subcutaneous malleolar bursa
- Retroachilleal bursa
- Retrocalcaneal bursa
- Flexor retinaculum
- Flexor hallucis longus tendon and sheath
- Superior extensor retinaculum
- Tibialis anterior tendon and sheath
- Inferior extensor retinaculum

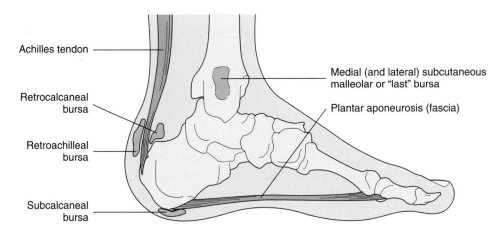

**FIGURE 7-5** **BURSAE AROUND THE ANKLE.** (From Hochberg H, Silman AJ, Smolen JS, et al., eds. *Rheumatology*, 3rd ed. Edinburgh, UK: Mosby, 2003.)

*Labels in figure:*
- Achilles tendon
- Retrocalcaneal bursa
- Retroachilleal bursa
- Subcalcaneal bursa
- Medial (and lateral) subcutaneous malleolar or "last" bursa
- Plantar aponeurosis (fascia)

tendon from frictional wear against the posterior calcaneus. The retroachilleal bursa lies between the skin and the Achilles tendon and protects the tendon from external pressure. The subcalcaneal bursa lies beneath the skin over the plantar aspect of the calcaneus. The medial and lateral subcutaneous malleolar, or "last" bursae, are located near the medial and lateral malleoli, respectively.

Movements of the ankle include dorsiflexion and plantar flexion (Figure 7-6). The axis of movement passes approximately through the malleoli. The gastrocnemius and soleus muscles are the prime plantar flexors of the ankle. The tibialis anterior and extensor digitorum longus muscles are the prime dorsiflexors.

### SUBTALAR JOINT

The **subtalar (talocalcaneal) joint** lies between the talus and the calcaneus and has three facets: *anterior, middle,* and *posterior.* Its tight capsule permits little synovial expansion,

about 30° of inversion (sole of the foot turned inward), and 10° to 20° of eversion (sole turned outward).

### MIDTARSAL JOINT

The **midtarsal (transverse tarsal) joint** comprises the combined talonavicular and calcaneocuboid joints (see Figure 7-1). The cuboid and navicular are usually joined by fibrous tissue, but a synovial cavity may exist. The midtarsal joint contributes to inversion (supination) and eversion (pronation) movements at the subtalar joint. It also allows 20° of adduction (foot turned toward the midline) and 10° of abduction (foot turned away from the midline). The axis of rotation of the subtalar and midtarsal joints is such that inversion is invariably accompanied by adduction of the forefoot, called *supination,* and eversion by abduction of the forefoot, called *pronation.* The tibialis posterior and tibialis anterior, aided by the gastrocnemius, invert the foot. The peroneus longus, peroneus brevis, and extensor

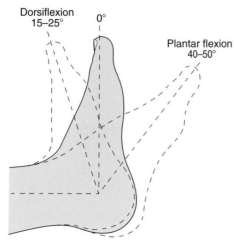

**FIGURE 7-6** ANKLE JOINT: NORMAL RANGE OF DORSIFLEXION AND PLANTAR FLEXION. (From Hochberg H, Silman AJ, Smolen JS, et al., eds. *Rheumatology*, 3rd ed. Edinburgh, UK: Mosby, 2003.)

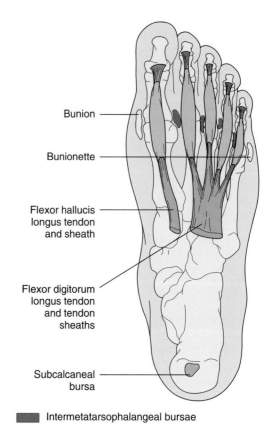

Intermetatarsophalangeal bursae

**FIGURE 7-7** PLANTAR SURFACE OF THE FOOT: FLEXOR TENDON SHEATHS AND BURSAE. (From Hochberg H, Silman AJ, Smolen JS, et al., eds. *Rheumatology*, 3rd ed. Edinburgh, UK: Mosby, 2003.)

digitorum longus evert the foot, aided by the peroneus tertius.

The **intertarsal joints** between the navicular, cuneiforms, and cuboid are plane-gliding joints that intercommunicate with one another and with the **intermetatarsal** and **tarso-metatarsal joints** (see Figure 7-1).

## METATARSOPHALANGEAL JOINTS

The **metatarsophalangeal (MTP) joints** are ellipsoid synovial joints that lie about 2 cm proximal to the webs of the toes. Their capsule is strengthened by the collateral ligaments on each side and by the **plantar ligament (plate)** on the plantar surface. The plantar ligaments are fused with the flexor tendon sheaths and are connected together by the **transverse metatarsal ligament,** which holds the metatarsal heads together to prevent excessive splaying of the forefoot. Small **intermetatarsophalangeal** bursae are frequently present between the metatarsal heads (Figure 7-7). The long extensor tendons form the **extensor expansions (aponeuroses),** which overlay the dorsum of the MTP joints and digits. The intrinsic muscles of the foot—including the flexor hallucis brevis, the lumbricals, the interossei, and the flexor digiti minimi brevis—are partly inserted into the extensor expansions and assist in plantar flexion of the MTP joints. The extensor hallucis longus, extensor digitorum longus, and extensor digitorum brevis dorsiflex the MTP joints. Movements at the first MTP joint consist of dorsiflexion (70° to 90°) and plantar flexion (about 35° to 50°). The other MTP joints permit about 40° dorsiflexion and 40° plantar flexion, as well as a few degrees of abduction (away from the second toe) and adduction (toward the second toe).

## INTERPHALANGEAL JOINTS

The **proximal interphalangeal (PIP)** and **distal interphalangeal (DIP) joints** are hinge joints. The plantar flexors are the flexor hallucis longus and brevis (great toe), the flexor digitorum longus (the lateral four toes at the DIP joints), and the flexor digitorum brevis (the lateral four toes at the PIP joints). The dorsiflexors are the extensor hallucis longus and the extensor digitorum longus and brevis, assisted by the interossei and lumbricals. The **digital flexor tendon sheaths** enclose the long and short flexor tendons, extending along the length of the toes to the distal third of the sole proximally (see Figure 7-7). A **bunion bursa** is commonly located over the medial aspect of the first MTP joint. Less frequently, a bursa is present over the fifth metatarsal head (**bunionette** or **tailor's bunion or bursa;** see Figure 7-7).

The PIP joints of the toes do not normally hyperextend, and plantar flexion is limited to approximately 50°. The DIP joints allow 10° to 30° dorsiflexion and 40° to 50° plantar flexion.

## ARCHES OF THE FOOT

The **arches of the foot** are the result of the intrinsic mechanical arrangement of the bones supported by ligaments and intrinsic and extrinsic muscles, particularly the tibialis posterior and anterior muscles. The arches of the foot act as shock absorbers during weight bearing. Each foot has two longitudinal and two transverse arches (Figure 7-8). The **medial longitudinal arch** is high and flexible and comprises the medial three rays digits—cuneiforms, navicular, and talus—and the calcaneus. It provides a resilient spring for weight bearing and forward propulsion in walking. The lateral two rays, cuboid and calcaneus, constitute the low, more rigid **lateral longitudinal arch.** The **anterior transverse metatarsal arch** includes the second, third, and fourth metatarsals

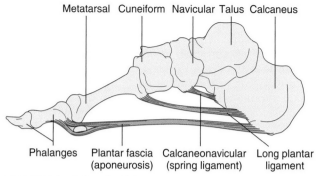

**Metatarsal  Cuneiform  Navicular  Talus  Calcaneus**

**Phalanges    Plantar fascia    Calcaneonavicular    Long plantar**
               **(aponeurosis)    (spring ligament)    ligament**

**FIGURE 7-8    THE FOOT: MEDIAL LONGITUDINAL ARCH AND LIGAMENTS.** (From Hochberg H, Silman AJ, Smolen JS, et al., eds. *Rheumatology*, 3rd ed. Edinburgh, UK: Mosby, 2003.)

| TABLE 7-1 | | |
|---|---|---|
| **PAINFUL DISORDERS OF THE ANKLE AND THE FOOT** | | |
| **Articular** | | |
| Arthritis | RA, OA, PsA, gout | |
| Toe disorders | Hallux valgus, hallux rigidus, hammer toe | |
| Arch disorders | Pes planus, pes cavus | |
| **Periarticular** | | |
| Cutaneous | Corn, callosity | |
| Subcutaneous | RA nodules, tophi | |
| | Ingrowing toenail | |
| Plantar fascia | Plantar fasciitis | |
| | Plantar nodular fibromatosis | |
| Tendons | Achilles tendinitis | |
| | Achilles tendon rupture | |
| | Tibialis posterior tenosynovitis | |
| | Peroneal tenosynovitis | |
| Bursae | Bunion, bunionette | |
| | Retrocalcaneal, retroachilleal, and subcalcaneal bursitis | |
| | Medial and lateral malleolar bursitis | |
| Acute calcific periarthritis | Hydroxyapatite pseudopodagra (first MTP) | |
| **Osseous** | | |
| Fracture (traumatic, stress) | | |
| Sesamoiditis | | |
| Neoplasm | | |
| Infection | | |
| Epiphysitis (osteochondritis) | Second metatarsal head (Freiberg disease) | |
| | Navicular (Köhler disease) | |
| | Calcaneus (Sever disease) | |
| Painful accessory ossicles | Accessory navicular | |
| | Os trigonum (near talus) | |
| | Os intermetatarseum (first and second) | |
| **Neurologic** | | |
| Tarsal tunnel syndrome | | |
| Interdigital (Morton) neuroma | | |
| Peripheral neuropathy | | |
| Radiculopathy (lumbar disk) | | |
| **Vascular** | | |
| Ischemic | Atherosclerosis, Buerger disease | |
| Vasospastic disorder (Raynaud disease) | | |
| Cholesterol emboli with "purple toes" | | |
| **Referred** | | |
| Lumbosacral spine | | |
| Knee | | |
| Reflex sympathetic dystrophy syndrome | | |

MTP, metatarsophalangeal; OA, osteoarthritis; PsA, psoriatic arthritis; RA, rheumatoid arthritis

and the heads of the first and fifth metatarsals. It becomes flattened on weight bearing but returns to its arched position when the weight is removed. The **transverse midtarsal arch** is more rigid and lies across the midtarsal region.

The longitudinal arches are held together by several layers of ligaments: the spring (calcaneonavicular) ligament; the long and short plantar ligaments that join the calcaneus to the metatarsal bases; and, most superficially, the **plantar fascia** (aponeurosis; see Figure 7-8). The plantar fascia extends anteriorly from the medial calcaneal tuberosity and splits at about the middle of the sole into five bands, one for each toe, to be attached to the transverse metatarsal ligament, the flexor tendon sheaths of the toes, and the proximal phalanges. The plantar fascia acts as a strong mechanical tie for the longitudinal arches by joining the three main weight-bearing points of the foot: the *calcaneus,* the *first metatarsal head* (including the two sesamoids), and the *fifth metatarsal heads.* During "toe off" in the later portion of stance phase, it helps the arch to reform and the foot to become more rigid.

## Differential Diagnosis of Ankle and Foot Pain

Ankle and foot pain may arise from bones, joints, periarticular soft tissues, plantar fascia, tendon sheaths, bursae, skin and subcutaneous tissue, nerve roots, peripheral nerves, or the peripheral vascular system, or it may be referred from the lumbar spine or knee joint. Static disorders caused by inappropriate footwear, foot deformities, or weak intrinsic muscles account for the vast majority of painful foot conditions. Table 7-1 describes the differential diagnosis of ankle and foot pain.

## Specific Disorders of the Ankle and Foot Region

### ACHILLES TENDINITIS

Achilles tendinitis usually is caused by repetitive trauma and tendon microtears due to excessive use of the calf muscles, as occurs in ballet dancing; track and field, including distance running and jumping; or from faulty footwear with a rigid shoe counter. Enthesopathy and insertional Achilles tendinitis may also occur in patients with ankylosing spondylitis (AS) or psoriatic arthritis (PsA). The tendon is a common site for gouty tophi, rheumatoid nodules, and xanthomas.

Clinical features include activity-related pain, swelling and tenderness over the distal tendon, and sometimes nodular thickening of the peritenon. Passive dorsiflexion of the ankle intensifies the pain. Two indicators that are often positive are the **painful arc sign** (movements of the tender, swollen area within the tendon with active dorsiflexion and plantar flexion of the ankle) and the **Royal London Hospital test** (tenderness on repalpation of a tender, swollen area within the tendon with the ankle in maximum active dorsiflexion and plantar flexion).

**Achilles tendon rupture** occurs most commonly in active young men, during a burst of unaccustomed physical activity involving forced ankle dorsiflexion or from intense athletic activities, particularly football, basketball, or tennis. It may also occur after minor trauma in elderly individuals with preexisting Achilles tendinitis, in patients with systemic lupus erythematosus or rheumatoid arthritis (RA) who are receiving corticosteroids, or after local corticosteroid injection near the Achilles tendon.

The onset is often sudden, with pain in the region of the tendon, sometimes a faint "pop," and difficulty walking. Swelling, ecchymosis, tenderness, and sometimes a palpable gap are present at the site of the tear. In partial tendon rupture, active plantar flexion of the ankle may be preserved but painful. In complete rupture, it is still possible to actively plantar flex the ankle by using the adjacent intact flexor tendons. However, the Thompson calf squeeze and the sphygmomanometer tests are positive, and rupture is typically associated with inability to perform a single-leg toe raise on the affected side. Abnormalities of the Achilles tendon can be confirmed by ultrasonography or magnetic resonance imaging (MRI).

**Retrocalcaneal, sub-Achilles, or subtendinous bursitis** is characterized by posterior heel pain that is aggravated by both activity and passive dorsiflexion of the ankle. Patients may develop a limp, and wearing shoes becomes painful. Tenderness on the posterior aspect of the heel, near the tendon insertion, is the main finding. Bursal distension produces a tender swelling behind the ankle with bulging on both sides of the tendon. Known causes include RA, PsA, and AS. Bursitis may also occur in association with both Achilles tendinitis and Haglund disease (abnormal prominence of the posterior calcaneal tuberosity, often associated with a varus hindfoot, causing chronic irritation of the Achilles tendon and bursa). When viewed from behind, a round, bony swelling can be seen just lateral to the distal part of the Achilles tendon.

**Retroachilleal or subcutaneous calcaneal bursitis,** also called a *pump bump,* produces a painful, tender, subcutaneous swelling overlying the Achilles tendon, usually at the level of the shoe counter, and the overlying skin may be hyperkeratotic or reddened. It occurs predominantly in women and is frequently caused by wearing improperly fitting shoes or pumps with a stiff, closely contoured heel counter.

## PAINFUL ANKLE DISORDERS

Ankle pain is a common patient complaint caused by a number of MSK disorders. Pathology in the bones, joints, ligaments, or tendons can all be accountable for pain and swelling in the region. The differential diagnosis can be narrowed by identifying the most affected side (medial versus lateral), by history, and on physical exam (Table 7-2).

**Ankle sprain** is one of the most common sports-related injuries. Most cases will heal spontaneously with supportive therapies. However, surgical management is often needed for two particular ligamentous injuries: a **deltoid sprain** with the deltoid ligament caught intraarticularly, with widening of the medial ankle mortice; and a **high ankle sprain,** with a widened inferior tibiofibular syndesmosis, causing real or potential widening of the ankle mortice.

## PAINFUL HEEL DISORDERS

**Plantar fasciitis** is the most common cause of subcalcaneal heel pain (Table 7-3). It results from repetitive microtrauma, which causes microtears of the plantar fascia at

---

### TABLE 7-2

### COMMON ANKLE PAIN BY ANATOMICAL SITE

**Lateral Ankle Pain**

Peroneal tendon injury/subluxation

Ligamentous injury (anterior and posterior talofibular ligament, calcaneofibular ligament)

High ankle (syndesmotic) sprain (anteroinferior tibial fibular ligament)

Fracture (talus, distal fibular, Jones)

Fibular or sural nerve irritation

Achilles tendon injury

Subtalar joint ligament injury

**Medial Ankle Pain**

Tarsal tunnel syndrome

Posterior tibial tendinitis

Ligamentous injury (anterior/posterior tibiotalar, tibionavicular, tibiocalcaneal)

Subtalar joint arthropathy

Medial tibial stress syndrome (shin splints)

Malleolar fractures

---

### TABLE 7-3

### PAINFUL HEEL DISORDERS

**Posterior Heel Pain**

Achilles tendinitis

Achilles tendon rupture

Achilles bursitis: retrocalcaneal and retroachilleal

Achilles enthesitis (enthesopathy: AS, PsA)

Subtalar arthritis

Tarsal tunnel syndrome

Painful dorsal calcaneal spur (rare)

**Plantar (Subcalcaneal) Heel Pain**

Plantar fasciitis

Subcalcaneal bursitis

Painful calcaneal fat pad

Bone (calcaneal) lesions

    Fracture (traumatic, stress)

    Epiphysitis (Sever disease)

    Neoplasm

    Infection

    Painful plantar calcaneal spur (rare)

AS, ankylosing spondylitis; PsA, psoriatic arthritis

its attachment into the medial calcaneal tuberosity. Risk factors include repetitive trauma from athletic activities, occupations that entail excessive standing and walking (e.g., "policeman's heel"), changes in footwear, reduced ankle dorsiflexion (< 10°), obesity, and pronated everted flat foot (pes planovalgus). It may also occur as an enthesopathy in association with AS or PsA.

Pain on the undersurface of the heel on weight bearing is the principal complaint. The pain is worse when weight is borne after a period of rest, such as in the morning, but eases on walking. Localized tenderness without swelling is present over the plantar surface of the medial calcaneal tuberosity. Passive dorsiflexion of the toes while everting the foot stretches the plantar fascia and often accentuates the discomfort. Radiographs may show a plantar calcaneal spur, which in itself is not the cause of the pain. Ultrasonography and MRI are useful diagnostic modalities.

**Subcalcaneal (infracalcaneal) bursitis** usually occurs in older persons as a result of repetitive trauma from improperly fitting shoes, falls, pounding the heel with some force, prolonged walking, or recent weight gain. Bursal distension produces a cystic swelling beneath the plantar aspect of the calcaneus. In contrast to plantar fasciitis, dorsiflexion of the MTP joints does not increase the discomfort.

A **painful calcaneal fat pad (painful heel pad syndrome)** is often confused with plantar fasciitis. The heel pad is normally composed of fibroelastic septa separating closely packed fat cells. Rupture of the septa in elderly, obese patients, during everyday activities or as a result of a sudden severe impact, results in attrition of the heel pad, poor shock absorption, and increased weight-bearing pressure on the calcaneus with reactive bony proliferation. Subcalcaneal heel pain occurs on weight bearing, with tenderness over the heel pad at the posterior weight-bearing portion of the calcaneus. This is in contrast to the more anterior and medial tenderness of plantar fasciitis. Radiographs may show reduction in the volume of the calcaneal fat pad and cortical thickening of the calcaneal tuberosity.

**Bilateral plantar and calcaneal traction spurs** are common in obese, stout, middle-aged and elderly individuals (Figure 7-9). Traction spurs are frequently asymptomatic, although heel pain may result from a coexistent plantar fasciitis, Achilles tendinitis, or painful heel pad.

**Flat foot (pes planus)**, or flattening of the longitudinal arch, is often asymptomatic but may result in muscle aching with prolonged standing or walking. Loss of the medial longitudinal arch on weight bearing and plantar displacement of both the navicular and the talus are the main findings. In severe cases, the calcaneus is everted (valgus), and the forefoot is abducted with a "too-many-toes sign" when viewed from behind. A callosity often develops over the prominent talar head, and marked wear of the soles of the shoes along the inner side is characteristic. Flat foot may be congenital or acquired, but **congenital flat foot** is more common and may be either hypermobile or rigid. In the hypermobile or flaccid flat foot, the arch is depressed with weight bearing but re-forms when weight is removed. The subtalar and midtarsal joints are mobile. In the rigid flat foot, there is abnormal fibrous, cartilaginous, or bony bridging between the talus and calcaneus or between the navicular and calcaneus (tarsal coalition). The medial longitudinal arch is absent in all positions, and subtalar movements are limited.

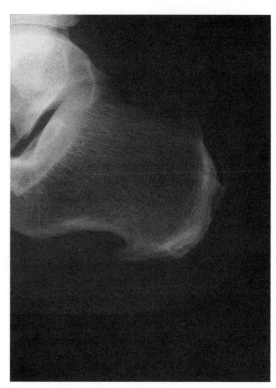

**FIGURE 7-9** **PLANTAR CALCANEAL SPUR.** (From Hochberg H, Silman AJ, Smolen JS, et al., eds. *Rheumatology*, 3rd ed. Edinburgh, UK: Mosby, 2003.)

**Acquired flat foot** may result from hypermobility syndrome, RA, neuropathic arthropathy, or trauma. Excessive weight and faulty footwear, superimposed on a mild congenital hypermobile flat foot, may also result in flat foot in adult life. Chronic tenosynovitis and rupture of the tibialis posterior tendon—the main dynamic stabilizer of the hindfoot against valgus (eversion) deformity, particularly in obese middle-aged women—can lead to a progressive asymmetric flat foot deformity or "collapsed foot." This is often associated with hindfoot valgus (planovalgus deformity) and forefoot pronation. Typically, the patient has difficulty standing on the tiptoes and ball of the affected foot while the contralateral foot is off the ground (positive **single heel-rise test**).

Acquired flat foot may be of three types: *mobile,* with the longitudinal arch depressed only with weight bearing; *spastic,* with spasm and tenderness of the peroneal muscles; or *rigid,* as with a collapsed foot fixed in eversion, known as a *hyperpronated foot.*

### Metatarsalgia and Morton Interdigital Neuroma

Metatarsalgia, or pain and tenderness in and about the metatarsal heads or MTP joints, is a common symptom with diverse causes (see Table 7-3). It often appears after years of misuse and weakness of the intrinsic muscles due to chronic foot strain from improper footwear, with the toes cramped into tight or pointed shoes. Pain in the forefoot on standing or walking and tenderness of the metatarsal heads and MTP joints are the main clinical findings. Plantar calluses and clawed toes are frequently present (Table 7-4).

## TABLE 7-4

### CAUSES OF METATARSALGIA

Chronic foot strain from improper footwear
Altered foot biomechanics: flat, cavus, or splay foot
Overlapping and underlapping toes
Interdigital (Morton) neuroma
Attrition of the plantar fat pad in elderly patients
Painful plantar callosities, including intractable plantar
    keratosis
Plantar plate rupture with secondary MTP joint instability
    (usually the second)
Hallux valgus, hallux rigidus, hammer and mallet toes
Arthritis of the MTP joints: OA, RA, PsA, gout, trauma
Bunion, bunionette, and intermetatarsophalangeal bursitis
Osteochondritis of the second metatarsal head (Freiberg
    disease)
Metatarsal stress (march) fracture
Sesamoiditis, sesamoid fracture, or osteonecrosis
Tarsal tunnel syndrome, neuropathy
Ischemic forefoot pain: peripheral vascular disease,
    vasospastic disorders (Raynaud disease)
Failed forefoot surgery

MTP, metatarsophalangeal; OA, osteoarthritis; PsA, psoriatic arthritis;
RA, rheumatoid arthritis

**Morton interdigital neuroma** often results from chronic foot strain and repetitive trauma caused by inappropriately fitting shoes or from mechanical foot problems, such as pronated flat foot or pes cavus. It represents an entrapment neuropathy of an interdigital nerve, rather than a true neuroma, typically between the third and fourth, or the second and third, metatarsal heads. The nerve is entrapped under the transverse metatarsal ligament or by an intermetatarsophalangeal bursa or a synovial cyst.

Symptoms include paroxysms of lancinating, burning, or neuralgic pain in the affected interdigital cleft and occasionally paresthesia or anesthesia of contiguous borders of adjacent toes. Relief of pain when the shoe is removed and the foot is massaged is characteristic. Walking on hard surfaces or wearing tight or high-heeled shoes increases the discomfort. The metatarsal arch is often depressed, and tenderness is present over the entrapped nerve, between the third and fourth metatarsal heads. The pain is made worse by compressing the metatarsal heads together with one hand while squeezing the affected web space between the thumb and index finger of the opposite hand (**web space compression test**). Injection of 1% lidocaine into the symptomatic interspace temporarily relieves the pain. Altered sensation may be found on the lateral aspect of the third toe and the medial aspect of the fourth toe. A soft-tissue mass (neuroma) may be palpable between the metatarsal heads. Movements of the adjacent toes may produce a clicking sensation due to shifting of the neuroma between the metatarsal heads, beneath the transverse metatarsal ligament (positive **Mulder sign**). The exact location of the lesion can be demonstrated by ultrasonography or MRI.

### Hallux Valgus

**Hallux valgus** refers to a lateral deviation of the great toe on the first metatarsal greater than 10° to 15°. It is more common in women and is often caused by a combination of genetic predisposition and the wearing of narrow, high-heeled, or pointed shoes. Other causes include congenital splay-foot deformity; metatarsus primus varus, an increased intermetatarsal angle greater than 9°, with or without metatarsus adductus of the adjacent second and third metatarsals; RA; and OA. Hallux valgus is often asymptomatic, but pain may arise from improper footwear, bursitis over the medial aspect of the first MTP joint (bunion), or secondary OA. As the first metatarsal moves into varus at its joint with the first cuneiform, its head also moves dorsally, resulting in a transfer of weight to the second metatarsal head. This is known as a **transfer lesion.** Altered weight bearing results in a callosity under the second metatarsal head with a hammer toe deformity and a flattened transverse metatarsal arch. If the deformity is marked, the great toe may overlie or underlie the second toe, and the sesamoids are displaced laterally.

### Hallux Limitus and Hallux Rigidus

**Hallux limitus** refers to painful limitation of dorsiflexion of the first MTP joint. **Hallux rigidus** is a marked limitation of movement or immobility of the first MTP joint, usually because of advanced OA. Intermittent aching pain, joint tenderness, crepitus, osteophytic lipping, and painful limitation of movement, particularly toe dorsiflexion, are common. Hallux rigidus usually occurs in elderly patients with OA, but it may occur after repetitive trauma, as in ballet dancing.

**Bunionette,** or **tailor's bunion,** is a painful callus and/or adventitious bursa overlying a prominent, laterally deviated fifth metatarsal head (metatarsus quintus valgus) and a medially deviated fifth toe. The pain is made worse by activity and by constricting footwear. It often occurs in conjunction with hallux valgus and forefoot splay. The intermetatarsal angle between the fourth and fifth metatarsals is greater than 10° (normal is 6.5° to 8°), and the fifth metatarsophalangeal angle is greater than 16° (normal < 14°). There is often exostosis of the fifth metatarsal head.

**Hammer toe** deformity most commonly affects the second toe. It is characterized by flexion deformity of the PIP joint, associated with dorsiflexion of the MTP and DIP joints (see Figure 7-11). A painful corn often develops over the dorsal prominence of the PIP joint. Leading causes include ill-fitting footwear—particularly narrow, high-heeled, pointed shoes—trauma, and RA, and it may also be a congenital deformity.

## Systemic Arthropathies Affecting the Ankle and Foot

### SPECIFIC DISORDERS OF THE ANKLE AND FOOT

#### Rheumatoid Arthritis

Rheumatoid arthritis can affect the hindfoot, midfoot, and forefoot (the most common site). Poor control will lead to joint destruction and deformities. Of particular concern is a rupture of the tibialis posterior tendon, which results in a collapsed midfoot with forefoot abduction and hindfoot valgus.

### Psoriatic Arthritis and Other Seronegative Diseases

Enthesopathy and synovitis affecting the ankle and foot region are often seen in seronegative arthritis. Dactylitis ("sausage toe") is considered a hallmark of this group of conditions.

### Gout and Other Crystal Arthropathies

Redness, swelling, and pain at the great toe MTP is the most common initial presentation of gout. The intense redness spreading into surrounding soft tissue can sometimes be confused with cellulitis. The midtarsal and hindfoot joints can also be affected by crystal arthritis.

### Osteoarthritis

The MTP joints, especially of the great toe, are frequently affected by osteoarthritis. Cock-up toes and hallux valgus and rigidus due to osteoarthritis are some of the most common foot problems.

## Physical Examination

### INSPECTION

The ankle and foot are inspected in both resting and standing positions for evidence of swelling, deformity, erythema, tophi, subcutaneous nodules, or ulcers. Abnormalities of gait are observed while the patient is walking. The gait or walking cycle can be divided into two phases: the *stance*, or *weight-bearing phase*, and the *swing*, or *non–weight-bearing phase*.

**Arthritis of the true ankle joint** produces a diffuse swelling anteriorly, obliterating the two small depressions present normally in front of the malleoli. By contrast, **ankle tenosynovitis** manifests as a linear swelling localized to the distribution of the tendon sheath extending across the joint. Swelling in the region of the Achilles tendon may be caused by tendon rupture, calcaneal bursitis, rheumatoid nodules, or urate tophi.

**Arthritis of an intertarsal joint** produces a diffuse swelling over the medial and dorsal surfaces of the foot. The exact location of the involved joint can be determined only by palpation. **Synovitis of the MTP joint** is associated with diffuse swelling on the dorsum of the forefoot that may obscure the extensor tendons. **Digital flexor tenosynovitis** produces a diffuse, tender swelling over the plantar aspect of the toe ("sausage toe"). Generalized swelling of the ankle and foot is common in edematous states.

In the standing position, the calcaneus normally maintains the line of the Achilles tendon. Normally, the middle of the heel is at 5° to 10° of valgus in relation to the middle of the calf. Deformities of the subtalar joint, which result in eversion (calcaneovalgus) or inversion (calcaneovarus) of the heel, are best observed from behind. Equinus and calcaneus refer to angulation of the ankle in plantar flexion and dorsiflexion, respectively. Inspection while the patient is standing may reveal lowering of the longitudinal arch (**pes planus**) or increased height of the arch (**pes cavus**).

The toes are simple extensions of the metatarsals. The first and fifth toes are often slightly deviated toward the middle of the forefoot. **Hallux valgus** deformity refers to a lateral deviation of the first (great) toe on the first metatarsal greater than 10° to 15° (Figure 7-10). Straightening or medial deviation of the great toe on the first metatarsal is called **hallux varus**, and **hallux limitus** refers to painful limitation of dorsiflexion of the first MTP joint. In **hallux rigidus,** there is marked limitation of movement or immobility of the first MTP joint, usually caused by advanced osteoarthritis (OA). **Cock-up** or **claw toe deformity** refers to dorsiflexion of the MTP joint and plantar flexion of both the PIP and DIP joints (Figure 7-11). **Hammer toe** refers to plantar flexion deformity of the PIP joint, usually associated with dorsiflexion of the MTP and DIP joints (see Figure 7-11). In **mallet toe** deformity, either the DIP joint is plantar flexed and the PIP joint is neutral, or the PIP joint is plantar flexed and the DIP joint is neutral. It is usually associated with a dorsiflexed MTP joint (see Figure 7-11).

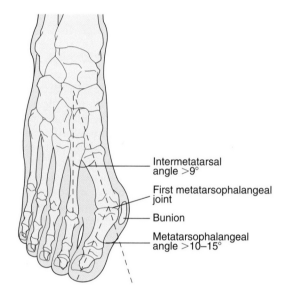

Intermetatarsal angle >9°

First metatarsophalangeal joint

Bunion

Metatarsophalangeal angle >10–15°

**FIGURE 7-10** **HALLUX VALGUS DEFORMITY WITH METATARSUS PRIMUS VARUS.** (From Hochberg H, Silman AJ, Smolen JS, et al., eds. *Rheumatology*, 3rd ed. Edinburgh, UK: Mosby, 2003.)

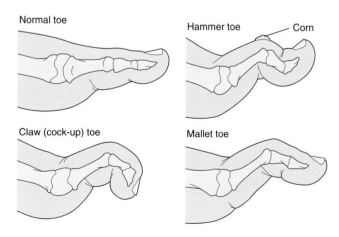

Normal toe    Hammer toe    Corn

Claw (cock-up) toe    Mallet toe

**FIGURE 7-11** **TOE DEFORMITIES.** (From Hochberg H, Silman AJ, Smolen JS, et al., eds. *Rheumatology*, 3rd ed. Edinburgh, UK: Mosby, 2003.)

## PALPATION

The ankle joint is palpated with the foot in slight plantar flexion. The joint is supported by the fingers of both hands, while the thumbs firmly palpate the anterior aspect of the joint (Figure 7-12). The capsule and synovial membrane are best palpated over the joint line, just distal to the lower end of the tibia and medial to the tibialis anterior tendon. The margins of a swollen synovium in other locations may be difficult to outline because of the overlying tendons. A **large ankle effusion** may bulge both medial and lateral to the extensor tendons and produce fluctuance: pressure with one hand on one side of the joint causes a fluid wave to be transmitted to the hand on the other side of the joint. **Ankle tenosynovitis** produces a superficial, linear, tender swelling that extends beyond the joint margins. The swelling is made more prominent by tightening of the involved tendon. Distension of the lateral and medial "last" bursae produces a localized, oval swelling over the anterolateral and anteromedial aspects of the joint, respectively.

A painful, tender heel may result from a number of causes. In **plantar fasciitis,** there is tenderness without swelling at the site of attachment of the plantar fascia to the inferomedial surface of the calcaneus. A **painful calcaneal fat pad (painful heel pad syndrome)** is associated with local tenderness in the center of the heel. **Subcalcaneal bursitis** produces a tender swelling on the plantar surface of the calcaneus. In **Achilles insertional tendinitis,** tenderness is present over the tendon near its insertion into the os calcis. **Retroachilleal bursitis** is characterized by a tender subcutaneous cystic swelling overlying the Achilles tendon. **Retrocalcaneal bursitis** produces a more diffuse swelling anterior to the tendon and posterior to the ankle joint. The subtalar joint is too deep to allow for accurate palpation, and effusion can rarely be seen on inspection.

The midtarsal, intertarsal, and tarsometatarsal joints are palpated by using the thumbs on the dorsal surface, while the fingers support the plantar aspect of the foot. Tenderness of the MTP joints can be assessed by gentle compression of the metatarsal heads together with one hand (**metatarsal**

**compression test**). Each joint is then palpated separately for tenderness or evidence of synovial thickening, using the thumbs over the dorsal surface and the forefingers over the plantar aspect (Figure 7-13). Chronic synovitis of the MTP joints often results in toe deformities, loss of the normal plantar fat pad under the metatarsal heads, callus formation, and **forefoot (metatarsal) spread** due to weakening of the transverse metatarsal ligament. The interphalangeal joints of the toes are palpated for tenderness, synovial thickening, or effusion using the thumbs and forefingers of both hands.

## RANGE OF MOTION

Ankle movements are tested with the knee flexed. The normal range is 15° to 25° of dorsiflexion from the neutral position, with the foot at a right angle to leg, and 40° to 50° of plantar flexion (see Figure 7-6).

Subtalar movements are examined with the ankle in the neutral position. The heel is grasped with one hand, while the other hand stabilizes the distal leg (Figure 7-14). The heel is then turned inward (inversion) to 30° and outward (eversion) to 20°.

To test movements of the midtarsal joint, the talus and calcaneus are stabilized with one hand, while the other hand rotates the forefoot inward (inversion) to 30° and outward (eversion) to 20° (Figure 7-15).

Movements of the first MTP include 70° to 90° dorsiflexion and 35° to 50° plantar flexion. The other MTP joints permit 40° each of dorsiflexion and plantar flexion. The PIP joints allow 50° plantar flexion. The DIP joints permit 10° to 30° dorsiflexion and 40° to 50° plantar flexion.

## SPECIAL MANEUVERS

In **tarsal tunnel syndrome,** the **Tinel sign** is positive if percussion of the posterior tibial nerve—found immediately behind the posterior tibial artery at the flexor retinaculum, behind the flexor digitorum longus tendon—produces paresthesia in the distribution of one or more of its two branches (the medial and lateral plantar nerves). Similar symptoms

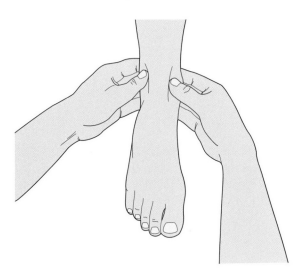

**FIGURE 7-12   PALPATION OF THE ANKLE JOINT.** (From Hochberg H, Silman AJ, Smolen JS, et al., eds. *Rheumatology,* 3rd ed. Edinburgh, UK: Mosby, 2003.)

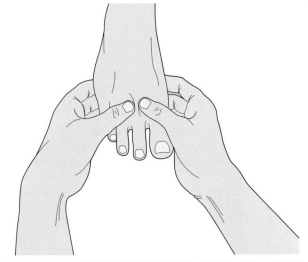

**FIGURE 7-13   PALPATION OF THE SECOND METATARSOPHALANGEAL (MTP) JOINT.** (From Hochberg H, Silman AJ, Smolen JS, et al., eds. *Rheumatology,* 3rd ed. Edinburgh, UK: Mosby, 2003.)

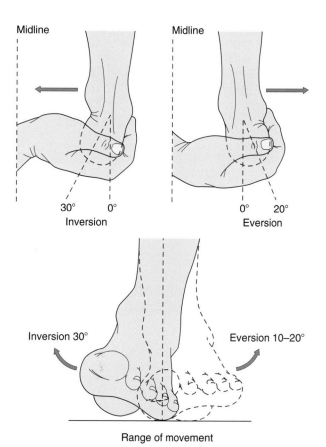

FIGURE 7-14    SUBTALAR JOINT: EXAMINATION AND RANGE OF MOVEMENTS. (From Hochberg H, Silman AJ, Smolen JS, et al., eds. *Rheumatology*, 3rd ed. Edinburgh, UK: Mosby, 2003.)

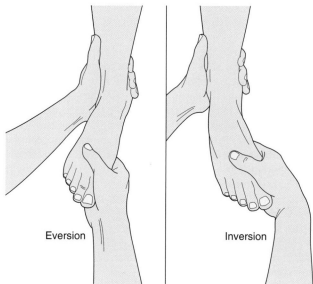

FIGURE 7-15    EXAMINATION OF THE MIDTARSAL JOINT. (From Hochberg H, Silman AJ, Smolen JS, et al., eds. *Rheumatology*, 3rd ed. Edinburgh, UK: Mosby, 2003.)

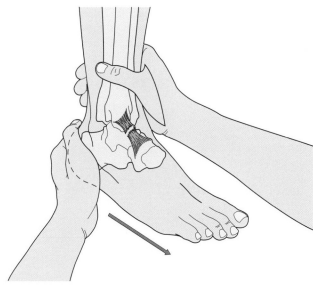

FIGURE 7-16    THE ANKLE JOINT: ANTERIOR DRAWER SIGN. A tear of the anterior talofibular ligament. (From Hochberg H, Silman AJ, Smolen JS, et al., eds. *Rheumatology*, 3rd ed. Edinburgh, UK: Mosby, 2003.)

can sometimes be induced by simple pressure on the nerve beneath the flexor retinaculum. Inflating a sphygmomanometer cuff around the leg to produce venous congestion may also reproduce the paresthesia (positive tourniquet test). In **anterior tarsal tunnel syndrome,** the deep peroneal nerve, which travels with the dorsalis pedis artery, is entrapped under the extensor retinaculum, and the Tinel sign is often positive.

Inversion and eversion sprains of the ankle can result in tears of the lateral and medial ligaments, respectively. Inversion sprains are more common and result in a tear of the lateral ligament, particularly its anterior talofibular band. To test the ligament, the distal tibia and fibula are held in one hand, while the calcaneus and talus are drawn forward by the other hand (Figure 7-16). A major tear of the anterior talofibular ligament allows forward movement of the talus on the tibia (positive **anterior drawer sign**).

In partial **Achilles tendon rupture,** active plantar flexion of the ankle may be preserved but painful. In complete rupture, it is still possible to actively plantar flex the ankle with the adjacent intact flexor tendons; however, gentle squeezing of the calf muscles with the patient lying prone, sitting, or kneeling on a chair produces little or no passive ankle plantar flexion (positive **Thompson calf squeeze test**). If the Thompson test is equivocal, a sphygmomanometer cuff is inflated to 100 mm Hg around the calf with the patient lying prone and the knee 90° flexed. If the tendon is intact, the pressure rises

to about 140 mm Hg with passive dorsiflexion of the ankle; but if the tendon is ruptured, the pressure changes very little (positive **sphygmomanometer test**). Rupture is typically associated with the inability to perform a single-leg toe raise on the affected side. In deep venous thrombosis of the calf, passive dorsiflexion of the ankle with the patient lying supine causes calf pain (positive **Homan sign**).

## Injections of the Ankle and Foot

The **ankle joint** can be injected via an anteromedial approach with the joint slightly plantar flexed. The needle is inserted at a point just medial to the tibialis anterior tendon and distal to the lower margin of the tibia. The needle is directed posteriorly and laterally to a depth of about 1 to 2 cm (Figure 7-17).

For injection of the **subtalar joint,** the patient lies supine with the leg–foot angle at 90°. The needle is inserted horizontally into the subtalar joint, just inferior to the tip of the lateral malleolus at a point just proximal to the sinus tarsi (the depression between the lateral talus and the calcaneus, in which lies the extensor digitorum brevis; Figure 7-18). Injection of the other **intertarsal** and the **tarsometatarsal joints** often requires fluoroscopic or computed tomographic (CT) guidance.

The **metatarsophalangeal joint** can be entered via a dorsomedial or dorsolateral route (Figure 7-19). The joint space is first identified, and then a 27 gauge needle is inserted on either side of the extensor tendon to a depth of 2 to 4 mm. Slight traction on the toe facilitates entry. The toe **PIP and DIP joints** may be entered in a similar fashion via a dorsomedial or dorsolateral route.

For **injection of plantar fasciitis,** the patient lies supine, and the point of maximal tenderness under the heel is marked. After infiltration with 1% lidocaine, the needle is inserted through the thinner skin of the medial side of the heel and advanced, in a lateral and slightly upward and posterior direction, toward the medial calcaneal tuberosity (Figure 7-20). The injection is made as close as possible to the plantar surface of the calcaneus. If the bone is struck,

the needle is withdrawn slightly before the corticosteroid-lidocaine mixture is injected.

For **injection of the toe flexor digital tendon sheath,** the patient lies supine, and a 27 gauge needle is inserted tangentially into the center of the flexor digital sheath, opposite the plantar surface of the metatarsal head (Figure 7-21). The needle is advanced slowly until gentle passive movements

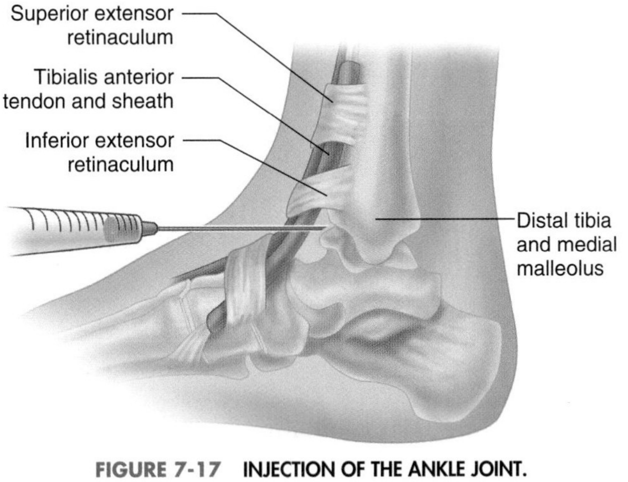

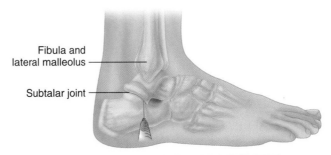

Fibula and lateral malleolus

Subtalar joint

**FIGURE 7-18    INJECTION OF THE SUBTALAR JOINT.**

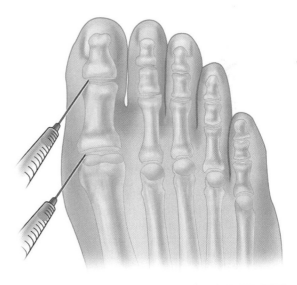

**FIGURE 7-19    INJECTION OF THE METATARSOPHALANGEAL (MTP) JOINT.**

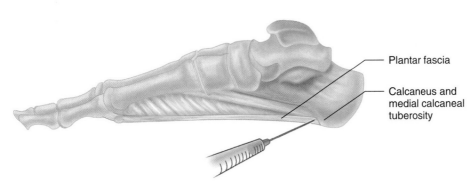

Superior extensor retinaculum

Tibialis anterior tendon and sheath

Inferior extensor retinaculum

Distal tibia and medial malleolus

**FIGURE 7-17    INJECTION OF THE ANKLE JOINT.**

Plantar fascia

Calcaneus and medial calcaneal tuberosity

**FIGURE 7-20    INJECTION OF PLANTAR FASCIITIS.**

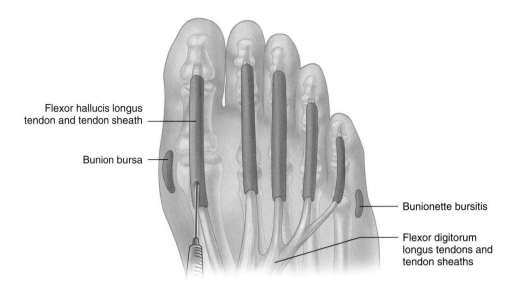

Flexor hallucis longus tendon and tendon sheath

Bunion bursa

Bunionette bursitis

Flexor digitorum longus tendons and tendon sheaths

**FIGURE 7-21    INJECTION OF THE TOE FLEXOR DIGITAL TENDON SHEATH.**

of the toe makes a crepitant sensation, indicating that the needle tip is rubbing against the surface of the tendon. When this occurs, the needle is withdrawn 0.5 to 1.0 mm before the corticosteroid is injected.

## SELECTED READINGS

Bottger, B.A., Schweitzer, M.E., El-Noueam, K., Desai, M., 1998. MR imaging of the normal and abnormal retrocalcaneal bursae. Am. J. Roentgenol. 170, 1239–1241.

Fam, A.G., 2003. The ankle and foot. In: Hochberg, H., Silman, A.J., Smolen, J.S. (Eds.), Rheumatology, third ed. Mosby, Edinburgh, UK, pp. 681–692.

Gould, J.S., 1989. Metatarsalgia. Orthop. Clin. North Am. 20, 553–562.

Maffulli, N., 1999. Rupture of the Achilles tendon. J. Bone Joint Surg. Am. 81, 1019–1035.

Mazzone, M.F., McCue, T., 2002. Common conditions of the Achilles tendon. Am. Fam. Physician 65, 1805–1810.

Perry, J., 1983. Anatomy and biomechanics of the hindfoot. Clin. Orthop. 177, 9–15.

Riddle, D.L., Pulisic, M., Pidcoe, P., Johnson, R.E., 2003. Risk factors for plantar fasciitis: A matched case-control study. J. Bone Joint Surg. Am. 85, 872–877.

Schepsis, A.A., Leach, R.E., Gorzyca, J., 1991. Plantar fasciitis: Etiology, treatment, surgical results and review of the literature. Clin. Orthop. 266, 185–196.

Stephens, M.M., 1994. Haglund's deformity and retrocalcaneal bursitis. Orthop. Clin. North Am. 25, 41–46.

Wu, K.K., 2000. Morton neuroma and metatarsalgia. Curr. Opin. Rheumatol. 12, 131–142.

# 8

# THE SPINE

George V. Lawry • Hamilton Hall •
Carlo Ammendolia • Adel G. Fam

## Applied Anatomy and Biomechanics of the Spine

The vertebral column consists of **33 vertebrae—7 cervical (C), 12 thoracic (T), 5 lumbar (L), 5 sacral (S),** and **4 coccygeal** vertebrae—and **23 intervertebral disks.** Its structure provides a remarkable combination of rigidity, stability, and flexibility. Rigidity provides an essential vertical bony axis, stability provides strong scaffolding for cavities and extremities, and flexibility permits complex movements of the neck and low back. The spinal column is composed of four **balanced curves:** a *cervical lordosis,* a *thoracic kyphosis,* a *lumbar lordosis,* and a *sacrococcygeal kyphosis* (Figure 8-1). The compensatory nature of the balanced spinal curves allows the normal resting, erect posture to be maintained with minimal muscular effort.

The vertebrae have important common features: an anterior, weight-bearing element, called the **vertebral body,** and the **posterior elements,** including the neural arch and facet joints. The vertebrae and vertebral bodies increase progressively in size from C2 to S1 and decrease from S2 to the fourth coccygeal vertebra.

The **neural arch** is made up of two **pedicles** attached to the vertebral body and two **laminae,** which fuse in the midline to form the **spinous process.** Three pairs of bony processes project from the arch close to the junction of the pedicles and laminae: two *transverse processes,* two *superior articular processes,* and two *inferior articular processes.* The paired articular processes at each level form the **facet (apophyseal) joints** (Figure 8-2). In the cervical spine, these joints bear about half of the weight of the head. In the lumbar spine, they accept less than a fifth of the load. This fact accounts for the relative difference in size between the facet joints and the vertebral bodies in the neck and low back. In the cervical spine, the joints are flat and slide easily. In the lumbar spine, they are curved to lock together and provide stability. In both areas the superior joints face backward.

Several vertebrae deserve special comment, because they have unique features. The first cervical vertebra, C1, also called the **atlas,** lacks a vertebral body and consists of anterior and posterior arches and two cup-shaped lateral masses (Figure 8-3). Just as Atlas in Greek mythology was forced to bear the world on his shoulders, so the cervical atlas (C1) bears the skull on its "shoulders" (lateral masses), each articulating with the occipital condyles on either side of the foramen magnum at the **atlantooccipital joints.** These joints allow nearly 40° of flexion–extension, for nodding the head, and 10° of lateral flexion. The second cervical vertebra, C2 or the **axis,** has a vertebral body anteriorly; from it a fingerlike peg projects superiorly. This bony process, called the **odontoid** or **dens** (*den* and *dont* from the Latin "tooth"), fits snugly against the anterior arch of the atlas, forming the atlantoaxial joint. The two are held together by the fibrous **transverse ligament,** which runs behind the odontoid process (see Figure 8-3). Rotation of the cervical spine, such as when shaking the head "no," occurs mainly at the **atlantoaxial joints** (about 50°). There are no intervertebral disks between the atlas and occiput or between the atlas and the axis.

The third through the seventh **cervical vertebrae** possess more typical vertebral bodies and posterior elements, as well as intervertebral disks, and a foramen in each transverse process for the vertebral arteries. In addition, C3 through C7 vertebrae frequently form bony projections posteriorly and laterally from the superior end plate of each vertebra, which articulate with the beveled inferolateral surface of the vertebra above to form the **uncovertebral joints** or **joints of Luschka.** They also provide lateral stability to the discovertebral complex and form a barrier to extrusion of disk material posterolaterally (Figure 8-4). The C3 through C7 vertebrae allow cervical spine flexion, extension, lateral inclination, and rotation.

The **thoracic vertebrae** have unique, long, posterolaterally directed transverse processes. A facet near the end of each transverse process articulates with the neck of the corresponding rib (**costotransverse joints**), and notches in the posterolateral aspect of adjacent vertebrae form articulations for the head of each rib (**costovertebral joints**). Movements of the thoracic spine are limited by the buttressing effects of the rib cage, the small size of the intervertebral disks, and the frontal direction of the facet joints. The superior thoracic facet joints face upward, backward, and slightly laterally.

The **lumbar vertebrae** are remarkable for their size. The larger cross-sectional area of the lumbar vertebral end plates facilitates load bearing by the intervertebral disks. The larger surface area of the lumbar facet joints provides increased torsional and sheer stability to these spinal segments, limiting rotation but allowing side bending. The superior facet joints face medially and backward (see Figure 8-2). The lumbar spine allows a greater range of motion (ROM) than the thoracic spine, including flexion, extension, lateral flexion, and rotation.

The wedge-shaped **sacrum** provides the inferior anchor for the spinal column, where it articulates with the posterior bony pelvis at the **sacroiliac (SI) joints** on each side. The **coccyx** consists of four small, fused vertebrae at the inferior end of the spinal column.

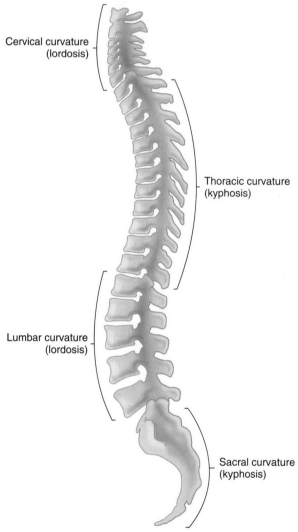

**FIGURE 8-1   VERTEBRAL COLUMN: FOUR BALANCED CURVES.**

Cervical curvature (lordosis)

Thoracic curvature (kyphosis)

Lumbar curvature (lordosis)

Sacral curvature (kyphosis)

## SPINAL JOINTS

### Discovertebral Joints

Each vertebral end plate is coated with a layer of hyaline articular cartilage (**cartilaginous end plate**). Adjacent vertebrae are united by a **fibrocartilaginous intervertebral disk.** Concentric, crossing layers of tough fibrous tissue, the **annulus fibrosus,** make up the outer circumference of the disk, enclosing a central, shock-absorbing gelatinous core, the **nucleus pulposus** (Figure 8-5). The intervertebral disks account for about one fourth of the height of the vertebral column above the sacrum. The sacrococcygeal vertebrae are fused and have no intervertebral disks. The disks are thickest in the lumbar spine and thinnest in the thoracic spine, and the cervical disks are intermediate in size. The intervertebral disks distribute the weight over the surface of the vertebral body and act as shock absorbers during loading, converting vertical load into horizontal thrust, which is absorbed by the elastic mechanism of the annulus. The disks provide a strong tie between the vertebrae yet allow a greater range of spinal movements compared with a solid column.

### Facet Joints

The **facet (apophyseal) joints** between the superior and inferior articular processes allow movement of the spine. The articulating facets are coated with hyaline articular cartilage, lined with synovium, and joined by a thin articular capsule.

### Sacroiliac Joints

The SI joints are irregular, narrow articulations that join the spinal column to the pelvis on each side and lend stability to the posterior pelvic circle. The anterior (ventral) and inferior part of each SI joint is a synovium-lined articulation, whereas the posterior (dorsal) and superior part is a fibrous joint supported by strong ligaments. There is little or no movement at the SI joints.

## LIGAMENTS

Numerous ligaments stabilize the anterior and posterior elements of the spinal column. The **anterior longitudinal ligament** is a strong, broad fibrous band that runs from

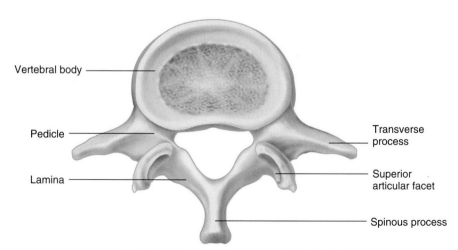

Vertebral body

Pedicle

Lamina

Transverse process

Superior articular facet

Spinous process

**FIGURE 8-2   LUMBAR VERTEBRA: BASIC ANATOMY.**

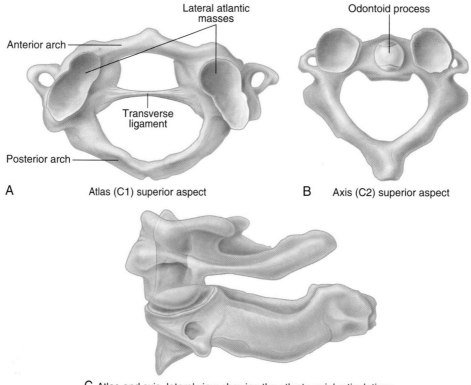

Lateral atlantic masses

Anterior arch

Transverse ligament

Posterior arch

A    Atlas (C1) superior aspect

Odontoid process

B    Axis (C2) superior aspect

C Atlas and axis, lateral view showing the atlanto-axial articulations

**FIGURE 8-3    ATLAS AND AXIS (C1 AND C2).**

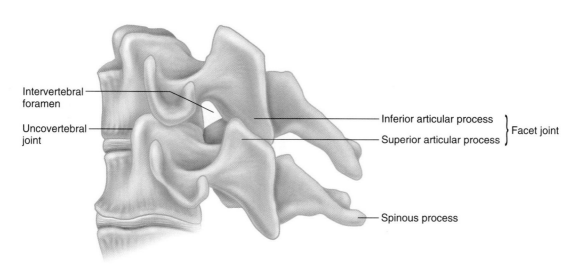

Intervertebral foramen

Uncovertebral joint

Inferior articular process ⎫
Superior articular process ⎭ Facet joint

Spinous process

**FIGURE 8-4    CERVICAL UNCOVERTEBRAL AND FACET JOINTS AT C5/C6.**

the occiput to the sacrum, where it anchors the anterior vertebral surfaces and intervertebral disks (Figure 8-6); it prevents excessive extension of the spine. The **posterior longitudinal ligament** also runs the length of the spinal column. It is a weak and narrow band but broadens where it attaches to the posterior intervertebral disks. Multiple ligaments also stabilize the posterior elements. The **ligamentum flavum** interconnects the vertebral laminae at the posterior roof of the spinal canal, and the weak **interspinous ligaments** and the stronger **supraspinous ligaments** interconnect the spinous processes. The latter two sets of ligaments partially limit forward and lateral flexion of the spine (see

Figure 8-6). The **intertransverse ligaments** interconnect the transverse processes.

## MUSCLES

A number of muscles span multiple spinal segments and provide both mobility and considerable stability to the spine. The cervical and lumbosacral spines are endowed with muscles anteriorly, laterally, and posteriorly, whereas the thoracic spinal muscles are exclusively posterior. Abdominal, trunk, and limb muscles assist the intrinsic muscles of the spine in achieving a wide range of movements.

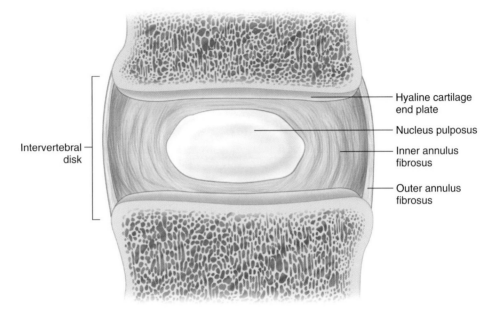

**FIGURE 8-5 INTERVERTEBRAL DISK.**

Hyaline cartilage end plate

Nucleus pulposus

Inner annulus fibrosus

Outer annulus fibrosus

Intervertebral disk

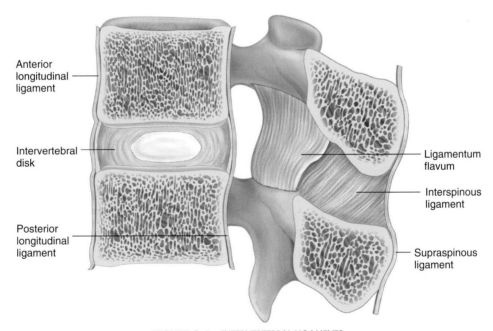

**FIGURE 8-6 INTERVERTEBRAL LIGAMENTS.**

Anterior longitudinal ligament

Intervertebral disk

Posterior longitudinal ligament

Ligamentum flavum

Interspinous ligament

Supraspinous ligament

## SPINAL STABILITY

The vertebral column, a modified segmented rod, is stabilized by both intrinsic (static) and extrinsic (dynamic) factors. **Intrinsic (static) stabilizers** include the intervertebral disks, the capsule of the facet joints, and various ligaments, particularly the anterior longitudinal and supraspinous ligaments and the ligamentum flavum. **Extrinsic (dynamic) stabilizers** include the paraspinal muscles (erector spinae, trunk, and abdominal muscles). Contraction of the trunk and abdominal muscles produces a rigid-walled cylinder in front of the spine. This transmits to the pelvis part of the forces generated on loading the spine and also acts as a lever that assists in reducing the load on the spine. The center of

gravity falls either through or 1 cm anterior to the L4 vertebra. Shock absorption and vertical loads on the spine are attenuated by the balanced spinal curves, intervertebral disks, and paravertebral and trunk muscles.

## SURFACE ANATOMY

Several landmarks can facilitate localizing specific spinal segments. The T2 vertebra is at the level of the top of the manubrium sterni. The apex of the spine of the scapula is even with the spine of T3, and the lower pole of the scapula is in line with the spine of T8. Although the position of the umbilicus varies with age, sex, obesity, and posture, it is generally on the same plane as the bottom of L3. A line connecting the upper border of the iliac crests crosses the midline at the level of L4, and a line drawn between the posterior superior iliac spines—beneath the sacral dimples, or "dimples of Venus"—crosses the second sacral segment.

## History and Physical Examination

An accurate and focused history is the essential first step in the diagnosis of patients with spinal pain. The information obtained from the history, which should include an assessment of possible risk factors for potentially serious underlying pathology, directs the subsequent physical examination and decision making regarding the need for additional tests and the choice of therapeutic measures to reduce the patient's pain and restore function.

Categorizing patients with spinal pain into one of **three broad groups** can be particularly useful both diagnostically and therapeutically. The groups comprise the three kinds of pain:

1. Mechanical, spine-predominant (neck or low back) pain
2. Neurological, extremity-predominant radicular (arm or leg) pain
3. Spinal pain associated with another specific etiology

### FOCUS OF INITIAL HISTORY IS CRITICAL

It is crucial to focus the initial history on the one problem that accounts for more than 80% of neck and back symptoms: **mechanical, spine-predominant (neck or low back) pain** (Figure 8-7). *Mechanical pain* can be defined as symptoms arising from the irritation of a physical element or elements within the spine, predictably aggravated and relieved by specific movements and positions. It is the result of an anatomic malfunction unrelated to infection, neoplastic disease, systemic illness, or major trauma. An additional 10% of patients may present with symptoms of nerve root irritation with **neurological, extremity-predominant radicular (arm or leg) pain.**

The overwhelming clinical probability that there is a purely structural pain generator involved in the patient's neck or back pain makes it logical to begin the history by attempting to recognize a clearly defined mechanical pattern. Although spinal pain can arise from a myriad sources, the patient's presenting symptoms are critical to understanding the clinical problem and should be obtained in a systematic and consistent manner.

## History

### ESSENTIAL INITIAL QUESTIONS

**"Where exactly is your pain the worst?"** The interrogation is precise, because the patient's response must separate axial pain, along the spine, from pain primarily in the extremities. Although the pain may be referred into the arms or legs, mechanical pain usually remains most intense around the axial skeleton. In contrast, pain felt more strongly in the limbs than in the neck or back is usually radicular, representing direct nerve root irritation and typically traveling along the course of the involved roots.

Making identification even more problematic is the fact that mechanical neck or back pain is not necessarily felt mainly in the neck or back. Referred pain that originates in the neck can be most intense along the trapezius ridge; the interscapular region; at the occiput, sometimes with headache extending to the retroorbital area; and along the jaw line or the anterior chest (cervical angina). Referred pain that originates in the back may be perceived as most excruciating in the buttocks, groin, flanks, or trochanters.

**"Is your pain constant or intermittent?"** Over time, individual episodes of pain can blend into an unbroken, painful continuum. Some patients may be reluctant to admit that their pain is intermittent for fear of minimizing its importance, so how this question is framed is critical. The most effective way to introduce the question is to set the parameters before the patient is given the opportunity to respond. Acknowledge that you understand that the pain is severe and likely to recur before asking if there is ever a time when it is gone. Inquire specifically about such things as "the best time of day" or "the activity most likely to give you relief."

**"When your pain goes away, does it disappear completely?"** The patient's description of intermittent pain should be verified with this follow-up question, because patients may qualify their first response by saying that although the pain is much reduced, they are never totally pain free. Uncomplicated mechanical pain is typically intermittent. Without periods of total freedom from pain, decreased symptoms do not qualify as intermittent pain; the symptoms must be regarded as constant.

### NECESSARY INFORMATION

Taking a history of spinal pain should be directed yet comprehensive. Appropriate evaluation requires a careful delineation of pain characteristics and associated features. A helpful mnemonic for characterizing spinal pain is **OPQRSTU**: O = onset; P = precipitating/ameliorating factors or prior episodes/treatment; Q = quality; R = radiation; S = severity; T = timing; and U = urinary or upper motor neuron symptoms.

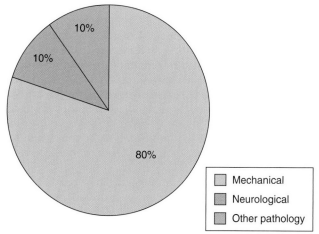

**FIGURE 8-7** **CHART SHOWING PERCENTAGES OF MECHANICAL, NEUROLOGICAL, AND PATHOLOGICAL SPINE PAIN IN PATIENTS.**

Information about the **onset, quality,** and **radiation** of the symptoms may offer clues regarding the source of the pain. Identifying **activities that heighten or diminish the pain** may offer insight into the nature or location of a structural problem and may point to a possible treatment strategy. Because neck and back pain are frequently recurrent complaints, much can be learned from a detailed account of any **previous episodes.** These may forecast the characteristics of the present attack. Ascertain the effect of **prior treatment.** If the current situation is similar to the last one, what worked before may well work again. The reported **intensity** of the pain is typically of little diagnostic significance but does give a measure of the patient's anguish and can serve as a baseline against which to measure future progress. Inquiries concerning changes in **bowel or bladder function** are mandatory with all patients. The history may uncover alterations in **neurological status** that must be investigated in the physical examination.

Finally, the history should establish the patient's **level of disability.** The question, "Because of your pain, what can't you do now that you were able to do before?" can elicit the degree of functional limitation. The intensity of treatment, indeed the need to treat at all, depends upon the answer.

*NOTE:* The lack of a defined mechanical response combined with a complaint of constant pain shifts the thrust of the questioning toward other nonstructural, potentially more serious etiologies. Questions should be directed at features associated with malignancy, infection, underlying visceral or systemic disease, psychosocial distress, or major injury. A group of important risk factors must be reviewed (see History and Physical Examination: Nonmechanical and Nonradicular Spinal Pain).

# Physical Examination

The physical examination of the neck or back should not be an isolated exercise. Its focus and, to some extent, its composition are determined by the history. Its principal purpose is to confirm or refute the hypotheses generated by listening to the patient's story.

## GENERAL EXAMINATION

**Observation:** The patient's general appearance, posture, and level of distress should be noted at the start of the interview. Watching the patient's gait, ease of movement, ability to sit without obvious discomfort, and facility in shifting from standing to sitting to a recumbent position provides valuable information.

With the patient suitably draped and the back exposed, inspect the skin over the spine for anatomic abnormalities, discoloration, superficial masses, and scars. Deformity or asymmetries can be recorded but should be considered significant only if they are unequivocal. Subtle alterations in alignment are rarely clinically important.

**Palpation:** Attempting to feel the bony prominences of the spine through the overlying skin, fat, fascia, and muscle is of limited usefulness. Depending on the size of the patient, it may be possible to approximate the locations of some of the vertebral spinous processes, particularly over the thoracic spine, but no other deep structures can be reliably identified. In the resting neutral position, the spinous processes of C7 and/or T1 are readily palpable in the midline at the base of the neck. Rarely in the lower lumbar spine it is possible to detect a step defect due to a high-grade spondylolisthesis (forward slip of one vertebra over the vertebra below), or an absent spinous process (spina bifida). Palpation can elicit areas of increased temperature, swelling, tenderness, or regions of painful, localized muscle tension. The relevance of these findings is usually determined by the history.

**Movement:** The normal range of spinal movement is a function of age, sex, body mass, and physical condition. Precise measurement is difficult, and wide variations in accepted normal values make the effort of little practical value. Of far greater clinical significance are the rhythm and symmetry of movement and the reproduction of the patient's usual pain as reported in the history. Uninhibited spinal movement is a smooth segmental progression; interference produces a consistent, unilateral shift or a block to flexion or extension that forces compensatory movements in the adjacent spine or large joints. Rotation and side bending are coupled movements (one cannot be carried out without the other) and should be about equal on each side. Ask every patient who exhibits a reduction in range of movement or an alteration in spinal rhythm whether attempting to move reproduces their typical pain.

## CERVICAL SPINE (Table 8-1)

**Inspection:** Assess the position of the head over the shoulders. Most patients with chronic neck complaints have a head-forward posture that is accentuated in sitting and noticeably reduced when the patient stands. In its middle position, the cervical spine should be in lordosis.

An assessment of the shoulder should be part of every complete neck examination. Neck posture has a significant effect on the range of shoulder movement.

**Movement:** Assess cervical flexion, extension, rotation, and lateral bending, and ask the patient about any reproduction of the typical pain during movement. Assess shoulder range of motion.

### Neurologic Examination

*Irritative tests.* Because of the mobility and multiple branches of the brachial plexus, the validity of irritative tests in the cervical spine to identify nerve root irritation is less certain than for those in the lower back. Rotating the head toward the painful side while forcing the neck into extension (Spurling maneuver, Figure 8-8) may reproduce the patient's described arm pain, but a negative test does not rule out direct root involvement. Extending, abducting, and externally rotating the arm while extending the wrist and tilting the head to the contralateral side may also reproduce radicular symptoms. The intervening brachial plexus significantly diminishes the test's sensitivity. Patients who experience a reduction in their arm pain by sitting with the hand on the affected side on top of their head (abduction relief sign, Figure 8-9) may be diminishing nerve root irritation by reducing tension on the lower plexus or lower cervical roots.

*Conductive tests.* Motor testing is the most reliable physical measure of nerve conduction. In order, the most commonly involved nerve roots in the cervical spine are C6, C7, and C5. The examiner should gauge the strength of elbow flexion (C6, biceps), forward elevation of the arm (C6, anterior deltoid), elbow extension (C7, triceps), finger extension

**TABLE 8-1**

## EXAMINATION OF THE CERVICAL SPINE

**Basic Examination**

*Observation*

Observe posture, movement, and behaviors

*Inspection*

Note resting posture and alignment, both sitting and standing
Inspect skin anteriorly and posteriorly

*Palpation*

Palpate occiput and spinous processes
Check for fibromyalgia tender points (suboccipital muscle insertions, medial upper border of trapezius, supraspinatus, and medial scapular borders)

*Range of Motion*

Cervical spine flexion, extension, right and left rotation, and right and left lateral flexion

**Special Testing: Suspected Shoulder Pathology (Neck and Proximal Arm Pain)**

Examination of shoulders

**Special Testing: Suspected Nerve Root Compression**

*Reflexes:* biceps (C5), brachioradialis (C6), and triceps (C7)
*Muscle strength:* deltoid, resisted shoulder abduction (C5); biceps, resisted elbow flexion (C6); triceps, resisted elbow extension (C7); interosseous, resisted finger abduction (C8)
*Sensation:* over lateral deltoid (C5), at thumb and index finger (C6), at middle finger (C7), and at ring and little fingers (C8)
*Spurling sign:* reproduction of radicular pain by applying gentle, firm pressure to occiput during combined rotation and extension to the affected side
*Abduction relief sign:* relief of radicular pain with placing distal forearm/wrist of affected upper extremity on occiput

**Special Testing: Suspected Myelopathy**

*Hoffman sign:* flick tip of middle finger; note involuntary flexion of thumb and index finger together
*Knee and ankle reflexes* and *ankle clonus*
*Babinski sign*
*Gait:* note broad base or unsteadiness, check

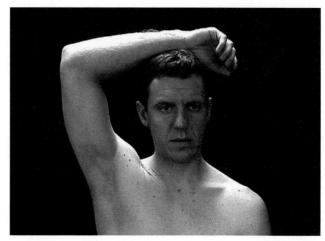

**FIGURE 8-9    ABDUCTION RELIEF SIGN (SHOULDER ABDUCTION SIGN).**

at the MCP joints (C7, extensor digitorum), and abduction of the arm (C5, central deltoid).

Reflex changes are identified by side-to-side comparison. The arms should be relaxed and supported. The biceps reflex is C5, C6; the brachioradialis reflex is C6; the triceps reflex is C7. Sensory testing is the least reliable investigation. The C6 dermatome includes the thumb, C7 covers the index and middle fingers, and C5 is best tested over the lateral deltoid.

***Upper motor tests.*** Involvement of the spinal cord can produce upper motor findings in both the upper and lower extremities. In the cervical myelopathic patient, flicking the tip of the middle finger will cause a sudden involuntary flexion of the thumb and index finger (Hoffman sign; analogous to, but not nearly as specific as, the Babinski sign in the lower extremities). In the lower limbs, cervical cord compromise can produce hyperactive reflexes, sustained clonus, and an extensor plantar response with an up-going great toe and spreading of the other digits (Babinski sign).

## THORACIC SPINE

### Inspection

Seen from behind, the thoracic spine should be straight. In the adolescent patient, a lateral curvature, usually convex to the right, is suggestive of an idiopathic scoliosis. This is frequently associated with a rotational deformity that distorts the symmetry of the rib cage and is best visualized by viewing the thorax from behind with the patient flexed forward at the waist. The curvature may be fixed or flexible and can be assessed by observing any change in the curve with side bending.

Seen from the side, the thoracic spine should exhibit a gentle kyphosis that balances the lordotic curves in the cervical and lumbar spines. Excessive kyphosis over the mid-thoracic spine or short segment angulation (gibbus) may indicate a developmental abnormality or old trauma with vertebral collapse.

### Neurological Examination

***Upper motor tests.*** The only possible neurological impairment that requires routine examination in the thoracic spine is spinal cord impingement. Individual root irritation produces focal pain around the chest that can be recognized on history but for which there is no corresponding physical

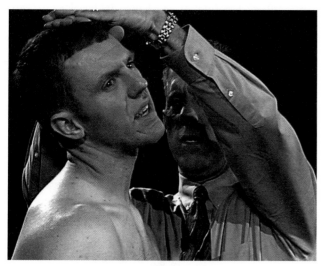

**FIGURE 8-8    SPURLING MANEUVER.**

test. Patients with suspected pathology in the thoracic spine should have their legs examined for increased reflex activity, clonus, and an abnormal plantar response.

## LUMBAR SPINE (Table 8-2)

### Inspection

When standing erect, the lumbar spine should be lordotic. The amount of lordosis is reduced with age, in structural abnormalities such as spondylolisthesis, and in ankylosing spondylitis. In the young, fit patient, the lumbar paraspinal muscles are easily visible as well-defined ridges running along the spine. Muscle wasting is common with advancing age and with reduced activity.

### Range of Motion

Assess lumbar flexion by instructing the patient to bend forward at the waist and attempt to touch the toes. Normal lumbar flexion should involve progressive reversal of the lumbar

| TABLE 8-2 |
| --- |
| **EXAMINATION OF THE THORACOLUMBAR SPINE** |

**Basic Examination**

***Observation***

Observe posture, movement, and behaviors

***Inspection***

Observe gait and heel and toe walking
Observe resting posture, alignment, and curvature
Inspect skin

***Palpation***

Assess skin tenderness to light touch or "skin rolling"
Palpate spinous processes (upper thoracic spine to sacrum)

***Range of Motion***

Lumbar spine flexion, extension, and right and left lateral
    bending

***Special Testing: Suspected Hip Pathology (Low Back, Buttock, and Proximal Leg Pain)***

Examination of hips

***Special Testing: Suspected Nerve Root Compression***

*Lying:* SLR
*Sitting:* Patellar (L4) and Achilles (S1) reflexes
Foot inversion and ankle dorsiflexion (L4), great toe
    dorsiflexion (L5), and foot eversion (S1)
"Quadriceps strength" (distracted SLR in sitting position)
Medial foot and ankle (L4), dorsum of foot (L5), lateral foot
    and ankle (S1) sensation
Perianal sensation, anal reflex, and sphincter tone (cauda
    equina syndrome)

***Special Testing: Suspected Psychological Distress—Waddell's Behavioral Signs***

Superficial or nonanatomic tenderness
Simulated rotation (pelvis) or compression (head)
Discrepant SLR (lying and seated)
Nonanatomic regional sensory or motor disturbances
Overreaction

***Special Testing: Suspected Visceral or Vascular Disease***

Abdominal, pelvic, and rectal examinations
Examination for abdominal aortic aneurysm and peripheral
    leg pulses

curvature from lumbar lordosis in the standing position to flattening of the lordosis in mid flexion to flattening or even slight lumbar kyphosis at the end of full flexion (Figure 8-10). Assess lumbosacral extension by asking the patient to bend backward. Simultaneously supporting the low back with one hand and one shoulder with the other hand provides stability and permits you to help the patient into full extension. Assess lumbar lateral flexion (lateral bending) by asking the patient to bend to the right and to the left. Place your hands on both shoulders and, if necessary, provide gentle pressure to help the patient into lateral flexion and assess the patient's response.

Note any abnormalities of flexion, extension, and lateral bending. Most importantly, note whether these motions reproduce the patient's pain.

An assessment of the hip joints should be part of a comprehensive low back examination. With the patient still standing, observe the pelvis from behind and identify the level of the iliac crests. Ask the patient to stand on one foot. Note whether the iliac crests remain level or whether the pelvis drops on the side opposite the standing leg. This pelvic "droop" (Trendelenburg sign) is a sensitive indicator of intrinsic hip disease and/or muscle weakness on the weight-bearing side. Repeat this test with the opposite leg.

Now ask the patient to lie supine and bring the hips into moderate flexion with the feet still on the exam table. Check for possible trochanteric bursitis by applying firm pressure to the lateral region of each trochanter, noting any tenderness. Next, check hip range of motion. Normal hip flexion brings the anterior thigh nearly to the chest. Return the hip and knee to 90° of flexion. Keeping the thigh perpendicular and the shin parallel to the examining table while testing hip rotation permits easy visualization of the arcs of movement. Hip external rotation is assessed by moving the ankle medially; hip internal rotation is assessed by moving the ankle laterally. Apply firm but gentle pressure to adequately assess range of motion. Question for the reproduction of typical pain.

*NOTE:* In patients with total hip replacements, be cautious in assessing hip range of motion. Avoid applying force when checking flexion and internal rotation, as this might dislocate the femoral component.

Pain originating from the hip joint itself is usually felt in the groin or medial thigh. Watch the patient's face while you perform hip rotation; a change in facial expression may be your first indication that hip range of motion is painful.

### Neurological Examination

*Irritative tests.* A passive straight leg raise (SLR) should reproduce the patient's typical leg-predominant pain resulting from irritation of the roots of the sciatic nerve (L4, L5, S1, S2). With the patient lying supine, support the heel of the foot on the patient's painful leg in the palm of your hand. With the patient's knee extended, lift the leg. An increase in the patient's reported leg pain constitutes a positive test (Figure 8-11). The location of the leg pain should be the same as that described in the history. *The production of back pain is not a positive test and does not indicate nerve root irritation.*

Many patients with severe sciatica cannot fully extend the knee on the affected side, and any attempt to do so will aggravate the characteristic leg pain. This constitutes a positive test. Patients demonstrating less nerve root irritability

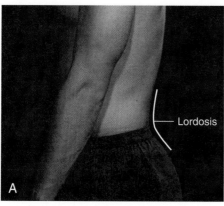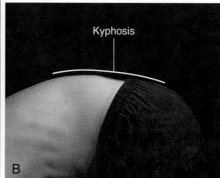

**FIGURE 8-10    NORMAL THORACOLUMBAR FLEXION. A,** Resting lordosis. **B,** Reversal of lordosis to slight kyphosis.

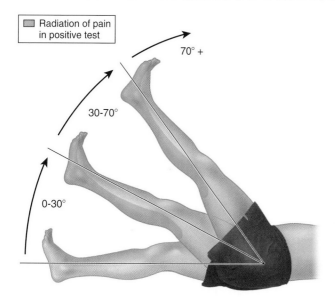

**FIGURE 8-11    STRAIGHT LEG RAISE.**

will allow increasing amounts of elevation. The higher the leg can be lifted, the less acute the radiculitis and therefore the less clinically significant the finding. But regardless of the point in the SLR at which the typical pain is produced, reproduction of the patient's specific complaint is a positive finding. Variations on the technique—such as dorsiflexing the ankle, applying pressure to the popliteal fossa, or passively extending the knee with the hip already flexed at 90°—are all intended to create the same leg pain. Once the examiner has exacerbated the patient's leg symptoms with one method, hurting the patient again in a different fashion seems unnecessary and unkind.

Occasionally, in cases of intense sciatica, performing an SLR on the unaffected leg will reproduce the typical pain on the symptomatic side. This form of crossed–straight leg test is the mark of an extremely irritable nerve root. It suggests a prolonged recovery and the likelihood that some type of intervention will be required.

A second type of crossed–straight leg test is far more ominous. In some patients, elevation of the affected leg produces not only the anticipated increase in the sciatic pain but also pain that radiates into the previously asymptomatic leg. This extremely rare finding can be the result of a large, centrally located disk herniation. Large, central protrusions are capable of compressing the entire cauda equina, including the lower sacral nerve roots (S3, S4, S5), which travel in the midline of the spinal canal and supply the sphincter muscles of the urinary bladder and the rectum. A massive central rupture of a lumbar disk (usually L3/L4 or L4/L5) can produce a cauda equina syndrome (CES) along with acute urinary retention with overflow and rectal incontinence. Decompression of an acute CES is a surgical emergency.

The femoral stretch test is comparable to the SLR but involves the roots of the femoral nerve (L2, L3, L4). With the patient lying prone, the examiner lifts the affected leg into extension at the hip (Figure 8-12). A positive response replicates the patient's typical anterior thigh pain. The maneuver must aggravate the leg symptoms described in the patient's history. Causing back pain is not a positive test.

***Conduction tests.*** Over 80% of the root involvement in the lumbar spine is either L5 or S1. Motor testing for L5 should include a Trendelenburg test (hip abductors, discussed earlier), ankle dorsiflexion power, and great toe extension. The muscles to be tested for S1 are the gluteus maximus (hip extensors), ankle plantar flexors, and flexors of the great toe. Less frequently affected nerve roots are L3 and L4, which control quadriceps power (knee extension), and L2, which supplies the iliopsoas (hip flexors).

The ankle reflex is subtended by S1. The hamstring reflex is supplied equally by L5 and S1 and is only useful for differentiating between those two commonly involved roots when it is compared to the ankle reflex. The quadriceps reflex is primarily L4.

Sensory testing is of limited clinical value but may be comfortingly confirmatory. The L5 dermatome covers the lateral side of the lower leg and the dorsum of the foot to the great toe. S1 supplies the small toes, the sole of the foot, and the back of the calf. The medial calf is L4.

The one place where sensory testing plays an important role is the saddle area. The skin surrounding the anus, including the midline between the upper buttocks and the genitals, is supplied by the same sacral roots that control bowel and bladder function. Reduced sensitivity to light touch in this region may indicate disruption of the lower sacral nerves and the possibility of an acute CES. When a cauda equina syndrome is suspected, a rectal examination to assess anal sphincter tone is mandatory.

***Upper motor tests.*** The spinal cord and the conus medullaris end at L2. No problem below that point can produce signs of upper motor damage. Some spinal cord lesions are

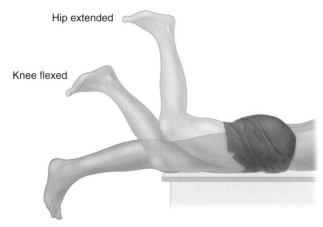

Hip extended

Knee flexed

**FIGURE 8-12   FEMORAL STRETCH TEST.**

capable of mimicking a single lumbar root lesion and can be completely missed without an upper motor examination. Finding sustained clonus or an extensor plantar response places the pathology at the cord level, above the lower lumbar spine.

## Nonmechanical and Nonradicular Spinal Pain and Other Etiologies

When the clinical picture is not a clearly defined mechanical or neurological syndrome, the focus must shift to identifying **risk factors** that suggest spinal pain associated with a possible serious underlying disease. A number of risk factors, or "red flags," have been shown to be associated with an increased risk of underlying serious disease—cancer, infection, or fracture—as a cause of spinal pain. These risk factors have been studied primarily in patients with low back pain, however they likely apply to spinal pain in general. These risk factors are listed in Table 8-3. Each serious disease is matched with several associated risk factors.

### CANCER, INFECTION, AND VERTEBRAL COMPRESSION

In patients with a history of cancer (excluding nonmelanoma skin cancer), recent unexplained weight loss, constant pain or disproportionate pain at night, age over 50, and failure to improve in 4 weeks increases the likelihood that **cancer** is the cause of the patient's low back pain.

A history of cancer, especially diagnosed within the past 10 years, appears to be the most important risk factor. The presence of this risk factor increases the probability of cancer as a cause of low back pain from 0.7%—the probability of *any* individual having cancer-related low back pain—to 9.0%, the probability of *this* individual having cancer-related low back pain, now knowing there is a history of cancer. In the *absence of a history of cancer,* the presence of any one of the other risk factors in Table 8-1 only increases the probability of cancer to 1.2%.

Spinal pain accompanied by fever, a history of recent infection (especially of the skin and the genitourinary tract), intravenous drug use, or immunosuppression are important risk factors for possible **spinal infection.**

| TABLE 8-3 | |
|---|---|
| **RISK FACTORS FOR POTENTIALLY SERIOUS DISEASE IN SPINAL PAIN** | |
| **Possible Cause** | **Key History and Examination Findings** |
| Cancer | History of cancer with new episode of spine symptoms |
| | Unexplained weight loss |
| | Disproportionate night pain or constant pain at rest |
| | Lack of treatment response |
| | Failure to improve after 1 month |
| | Age > 50 years |
| Vertebral infection | Fever |
| | Recent infection |
| | Intravenous drug use |
| | Immunocompromised |
| Vertebral compression fracture | Thoracic-dominant pain |
| | History of osteoporosis |
| | Corticosteroid use |
| | Minor trauma (in patients age > 70 years) |
| Spondyloarthropathy | Morning stiffness |
| | Improvement with exercise |
| | Alternating buttock pain |
| | Awakening with back pain during the second half of the night |
| | Onset age < 40 years |
| Visceral disease (referred pain) | Aortic aneurysm |
| | Pulmonary, cardiac/pericardial, GI, or GU disease |

Spinal pain in elderly patients with a history of osteoporosis or of corticosteroid use clearly raises the suspicion of possible **vertebral compression fracture.**

The **absence of any risk factors** listed in Table 8-3 for cancer, infection, or vertebral compression fracture provides the clinician with extremely high reassurance that these conditions are *not* likely the cause of the patient's low back pain.

### INFLAMMATORY SPINAL PAIN: ANKYLOSING SPONDYLITIS AND OTHERS

Spinal involvement in the **spondyloarthropathies** (e.g., ankylosing spondylitis and spondylitis with reactive arthritis or inflammatory bowel disease) may involve the low back, thoracic spine, or neck and tends to occur early in the course of the disease. Initial symptoms are frequently vague and often overlooked.

Characteristic features of inflammatory spinal pain include initial symptoms present before 40 years of age, an insidious onset, significant morning stiffness, improvement of spinal pain with exercise and worsening with prolonged rest, and a duration longer than 3 months. These features, although not specific, strongly suggest inflammatory back pain and are quite different from typical mechanical low back pain.

If the clinical history suggests possible inflammatory low back pain, a more focused assessment of the **sacroiliac joints** and spine is appropriate (Table 8-4). Ask the patient to lie supine. Bring one hip and knee into flexion as you cross the leg over the opposite leg and rest the patient's lateral malleolus

## TABLE 8-4

### EXAMINATION OF THE SACROILIAC JOINTS AND SPINE

**Special Testing: Suspected Sacroiliitis/Spondyloarthropathy**
*Lying*
FABER test (hip flexion, abduction, and external rotation)
Compress iliac crests

*Standing*
Schober test of lumbosacral spinal mobility

**Longitudinal Follow-up**
Schober test of lumbosacral spinal mobility: modified
  Schober (15 cm → ___cm)
Finger-to-floor distance in maximal forward flexion (___cm)
Finger-to-thigh distraction in maximal lateral flexion, right
  and left (___cm)
Chest expansion measured at level of fourth intercostal space
  (___cm)
Occiput-to-wall distance (___cm)

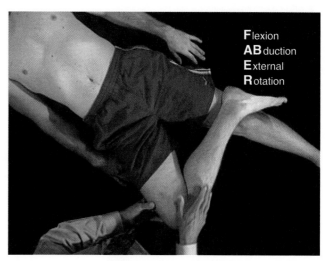

**F**lexion
**AB**duction
**E**xternal
**R**otation

**FIGURE 8-13   FABER TEST.**

on the opposite distal thigh (crossing the legs). Now, gently but firmly apply pressure to the medial aspect of the flexed knee, pushing it toward the exam table. This maneuver is called the *FABER test,* and it refers to the position of the hip in **F**lexion, **AB**duction, and **E**xternal **R**otation, stressing the ipsilateral sacroiliac joint (Figure 8-13). A positive FABER test requires reproduction of sacroiliac pain on the same side, felt in the upper inner buttock region rather than the lumbosacral junction, trochanter, or groin. This test may be difficult to interpret in patients with intrinsic hip disease, who may feel discomfort in the groin or gluteal region rather than the SI joint. Perform the FABER maneuver on the opposite side and compare.

Next, gently but progressively press downward on both superior anterior iliac spines, driving the iliac wings posteriorly toward the exam table. This maneuver stresses both sacroiliac joints, and a positive compression test requires reproduction of the patient's pain localized to the sacroiliac joint on one or both sides; induction of discomfort in other regions is not considered a positive test.

In patients whose history, examination, and imaging confirm the suspicion of a spondyloarthropathy, several **spondylitis-specific measurements** (Figure 8-14) are important to document initially, and in subsequent exams, to monitor disease progression and response to therapy:

The Schober test of lumbosacral spinal mobility in flexion
  (___cm)
Finger-to-floor distance in maximal forward flexion
  (___cm)
Finger-to-thigh distraction from neutral to maximal lateral flexion, right and left (___cm)
Chest expansion measured at the level of the fourth intercostal space (___cm)
Occiput-to-wall distance (___cm)

## VISCERAL DISEASE

Although relatively uncommon, a variety of visceral disorders can refer pain to the spine. Pulmonary, pleural, cardiac, and pericardial diseases may manifest with neck and shoulder pain. Gastrointestinal, pancreatic, genitourinary,

and atherosclerotic vascular disease (abdominal aortic aneurysm) may manifest with thoracic, flank, or low back pain. Inquiring about a significant pulmonary, cardiac, gastrointestinal, genitourinary, or vascular history may provide important clues to clarify the patient's "spinal" complaints.

## PSYCHOSOCIAL DISTRESS

When spinal pain persists, and serious disease has been ruled out, risk factors for underlying **psychosocial barriers to recovery** should be investigated. These include personal, social, and environmental factors (Table 8-5). Personal factors include attitudes, beliefs, emotions, and behaviors that the patient exhibits in response to spinal pain that are maladaptive and may prolong disability. Social and environmental factors pertain to how the patient interacts with his or her family, friends, and the workplace. Negative social relationships can impact pain perception and recovery. Psychological distress, the belief and fear that movement or activity will worsen the pain, and social isolation are other examples of psychosocial barriers that can delay recovery from spinal pain.

**Waddell's behavioral signs** were developed as a clinical assessment tool to help clinicians recognize important features of psychological distress and illness behaviors complicating low back pain. *They must be viewed in conjunction with the history and cannot be used in isolation as proof of illness behavior.* These signs are grouped into five categories of response:

- **Nonorganic tenderness:** superficial or nonanatomic tenderness
- **Simulation tests:** axial loading or rotation
- **Distraction tests:** discrepant straight leg raising
- **Regional disturbances:** "giving way" weakness or nondermatomal sensory disturbances
- **Overreaction:** inappropriate or exaggerated responses

The presence of significant superficial or nonanatomic tenderness, back pain in response to simulated axial loading or pelvic rotation, marked differences in response to supine and seated straight leg raising, nonphysiologic regional disturbances in motor or sensory function, and the presence of significant overreaction manifested by inappropriate

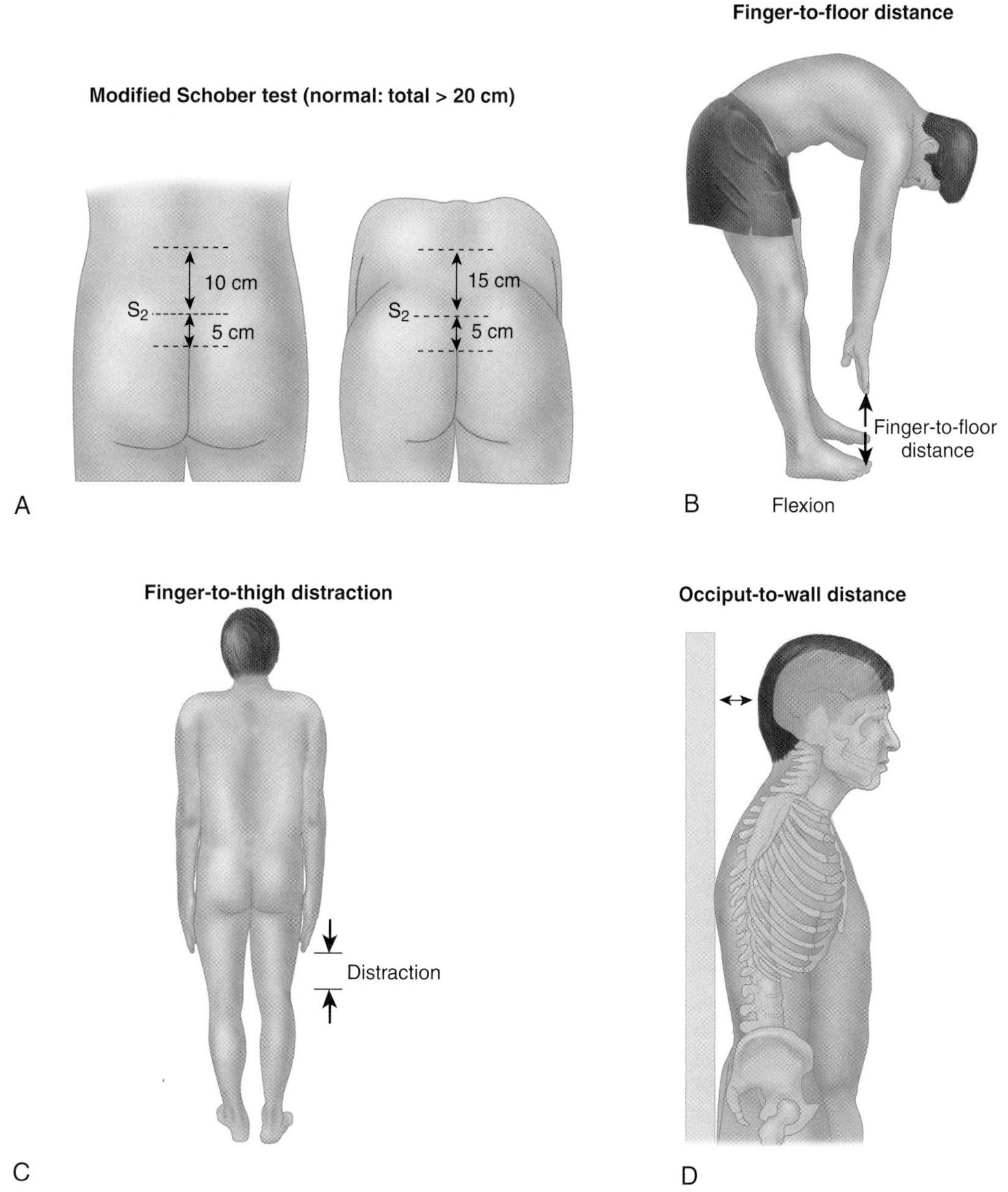

**Modified Schober test (normal: total > 20 cm)**

A

**Finger-to-floor distance**

B    Flexion

**Finger-to-thigh distraction**

C

**Occiput-to-wall distance**

D

**FIGURE 8-14**   **SPONDYLITIS MEASUREMENTS. A,** Modified Schober test. **B,** Finger-to-floor distance. **C,** Finger-to-thigh distraction. **D,** Occiput-to-wall distance.

**TABLE 8-5**

**PSYCHOSOCIAL RISK FACTORS FOR PERSISTENT SPINAL PAIN**

Poor overall psychological health
Fear-avoidance behavior
Emotional distress
Catastrophizing
Extremely high pain intensity
Depression
Anxiety, anger, or frustration in response to pain
Passive coping
Social isolation
Compensation/litigation case

guarding, limping, bracing, rubbing, grimacing, or sighing during the examination are important clinical signs and should not be ignored. The assessment of Waddell's categories can be readily integrated into a rapid, organized, and sequential examination of the low back.

The presence of **signs in three or more of Waddell's categories** may indicate significant psychosocial distress complicating the patient's low back pain. Overinterpretation of behavioral signs must be avoided. *Isolated behavioral signs should not be considered clinically significant.* Furthermore, the presence of behavioral signs does not rule out an anatomic problem.

Waddell unequivocally states that the presence of signs in three or more categories "simply shows the health care provider that abnormal illness behavior may be present as a coping strategy and that other learned cognitive and behavioral patterns and psychological influences may need to be addressed to improve treatment outcome (Waddell et al., 1980)."

## Imaging and Electrodiagnostic Tests for Spinal Pain

### IMAGING

The use of imaging in patients with spinal pain should be judicious and discriminating. Decisions should be based on the presence of clinical features (risk factors) in the history and physical examination that significantly raise the suspicion of underlying serious conditions. Specific causes of spinal pain that justify imaging include cancer, infection, fracture, spondyloarthropathies, and visceral disease (see Table 8-3).

No evidence shows that routine imaging for mechanical spine-predominant or neurological extremity-predominant pain (~90% of all patients with spinal pain) improves patient outcomes. In fact, in the case of low back pain, unnecessary lumbar spine imaging has been associated with poorer patient outcomes. In the absence of risk factors suggesting an underlying serious condition, current evidence recommends against the routine use of imaging—plain film radiography, magnetic resonance imaging (MRI), or computerized tomography (CT)—for spinal pain.

#### Cervical Spine

In the case of blunt trauma to the cervical spine, the Canadian Spine Rule or Nexus Low-Risk Criteria are useful for assessing the need for imaging to rule out serious injury, such as fracture or dislocation, in an emergency setting. In trauma patients presenting with severe and progressive neurological deficits, CT or MRI imaging is mandatory regardless of setting.

#### Lumbosacral Spine

For the detection of suspected cancer or infection, MRI and CT are more sensitive than plain film radiography. MRI is generally preferred over CT because it does not use ionizing radiation and is more sensitive for detecting pathology in the paraspinal soft tissues, vertebral marrow, and spinal canal.

Plain radiography should be considered for the initial assessment of high-risk patients suspected of vertebral fracture (patients with underlying osteoporosis or steroid use).

In the initial work up of patients presenting with signs and symptoms suggestive of spondyloarthropathy (see Table 8-1), plain film radiography of the lumbosacral spine and sacroiliac joints is recommended.

In patients with persisting low back pain and signs or symptoms of radiculopathy or neurogenic claudication, imaging with MRI (preferred) or CT is recommended only if they are potential candidates for surgery or other invasive interventions.

### ELECTRODIAGNOSTIC TESTS

Electrodiagnostic procedures are not a shortcut to diagnosis: they are a method of establishing physiological function. Evaluations may include peripheral **nerve conduction velocity** tests and/or **electromyography** to assess muscle activity. These investigations are most useful when they are used as part of a problem-solving approach to address a specific question arising from ambiguity in the clinical picture. They are best considered as an extension of a thorough physical examination and therefore unnecessary in patients with an unequivocal clinical presentation. *Electrodiagnostic testing is not part of a standard presurgical evaluation.*

## Common Painful Disorders of the Spine

### ACUTE, UNCOMPLICATED, MECHANICAL NECK AND LOW BACK PAIN

Acute, uncomplicated, mechanical neck and low back pain accounts for the vast majority of spinal pain seen in clinical practice. The clinical history is important, and with a mechanical presentation in the absence of radicular or serious underlying conditions, the diagnosis of acute mechanical neck or low back pain is acceptable. A definitive anatomic diagnosis cannot be established in up to 85% of patients presenting with acute low back pain. Up to two thirds have resolution of their symptoms in 4 to 8 weeks, although recurrences are likely. The same is true for nontraumatic acute neck pain. Fortified by this information, the clinician is able to direct subsequent management efforts at reassurance and resumption of normal functional activity and avoid extensive and expensive, and frequently misleading, imaging studies.

#### Acute, Uncomplicated, Mechanical Neck Pain

This is often referred to as *neck sprain,* although there may be no injury to the cervical spine ligaments. Patients may experience pain, from sharp to aching in quality, predominantly along the posterior or lateral spine from the occiput to T1. Associated pain often occurs in the occipital, interscapular, or shoulder regions with perhaps slight radiation to the upper limb. Pain may occur after minor trauma, athletic injury, or following awkward, repetitive, or static neck postures at work, during reading, or during overhead activities. Frequently, no clear precipitating event is evident, but inquiry should be made regarding occupational, recreational, or personal habits, such as computer and telephone use (computers, keyboards, head position, use of headsets), lifting and carrying (packages, car seats), and asymmetric loads (heavy handbags, book bags). A brief inquiry about sleep positions and pillow use may be helpful in delineating additional contributing factors.

Examination often reveals reduced ROM, diffuse tenderness, and spasm over the cervical spine, particularly suboccipitally. Whether pain originates in muscles, ligaments, disks, facet joints, or other structures is not clear and, given its often self-limiting nature is not usually clinically relevant.

#### Acute, Mechanical Low Back Pain

This is commonly referred to as *lumbosacral sprain,* although there may be no evidence of ligamentous injury. Acute low back pain is a common, usually self-limiting but frequently recurrent problem. The pain may be precipitated by lifting or bending, although in the majority of cases, there is no specific triggering event. It can be felt in the lumbar spine, lumbosacral junction, buttock, and posterior thighs and may occasionally radiate below the knees. Physical examination reveals diffuse lumbar spine tenderness, muscle spasm, and diminished ROM without radicular symptoms or signs. Whether the pain originates in the paraspinal muscles, ligaments, disks (annular tears), facet joints, or other structures is not clear and usually is not clinically relevant. Although up to 85% of patients may return to normal activities within 2 months, recurrences may occur in up to 75% of patients within 12 months.

## CHRONIC NECK AND LOW BACK PAIN

Neck and low back pain persisting beyond 3 months despite conservative management develops in a minority of patients and represents a significant clinical and economic problem. Chronic neck and back pain patients consume the majority of all expenditures for spine-related pain. Important historical features may relate to the patient's work, home, personal, and psychosocial history. Occupational risk factors associated with chronic neck and low back pain include physical stresses involved in manual labor, mental stress in both manual and office workers, and job-related stress due to lack of autonomy, lack of variation in workload, and lack of cooperation among workers. Pending litigation or disability determinations, marriage and family stress, drug or alcohol problems, and a history of anxiety, depression, or somatization are important contributing factors. These risk factors of chronic neck and low back pain identify patients who are at higher risk for persistent, disabling symptoms and permit earlier referral to multidisciplinary specialized centers (see Table 8-5).

## CERVICAL DEGENERATIVE SPONDYLOSIS

Degenerative changes of the vertebral bodies, secondary to cervical degenerative disk disease or uncovertebral and facet joint osteoarthritis, are referred to as *cervical spondylosis.* It commonly occurs in older individuals and is related to the loss of integrity of the intervertebral disk, secondary osteoarthritic changes in the uncovertebral and apophyseal joints, and hypertrophy and redundancy of the ligamentum flavum. Symptoms often involve local neck pain, sometimes with referral to the shoulders or scapulae. Stiffness and crepitus on motion, positional pain, and sleep difficulty may also be present. Physical examination may reveal tenderness and spasm, usually of the lower cervical spine, and reduced cervical ROM. Symptoms and signs of radiculopathy—and, less commonly, myelopathy—may also be present. It is important to note that the presence or degree of cervical degenerative spondylosis on imaging does not necessarily correlate with the presence or severity of neck symptoms.

## CERVICAL RADICULOPATHY AND MYELOPATHY

Neck pain combined with neurogenic upper-extremity pain strongly suggests cervical nerve root irritation. Pain may also radiate along the mid-scapular region. Far less common than uncomplicated mechanical neck pain, cervical radiculopathy usually results from disk herniation associated with

facet and uncovertebral osteophytes causing mechanical or chemical irritation of the nerve root and its dural attachment as it enters the neural foramen. Physical examination may reveal variable tenderness, paravertebral muscle spasm, and reduced ROM of the cervical spine. Neurologic testing may reveal diminished reflexes, strength, or sensation in the affected root distribution. Prolonged radiculopathy can result in muscle atrophy. Radiating pain can often be reproduced or intensified with manual cervical compression or distraction maneuvers. Thoracic spine pain with radiation around the ribs likewise suggests thoracic radiculopathy.

Acute or chronic neck or thoracic pain may be accompanied by a progressive loss of neurologic function due to cord compression (myelopathy). Both the spinal pain itself and the symptoms of myelopathy may be quite subtle. Changes in bladder or bowel habits, impotence, gait unsteadiness, and loss of small motor control in the hands are important signs of myelopathy.

## LUMBAR DEGENERATIVE SPONDYLOSIS

Degenerative changes in the vertebral bodies, secondary to lumbar degenerative disk disease and facet joint osteoarthritis, are commonly referred to as *lumbar spondylosis.* It typically occurs in older individuals and is related to intervertebral disk degeneration and osteoarthritic changes in the lower lumbosacral facet joints and sometimes to degenerative spondylolisthesis. Chronic low back pain with radiation to the buttocks is the most common symptom. The pain is mechanical in quality and is typically aggravated with activity and relieved by rest. Relatively brief morning stiffness, positional pain, and sleep difficulties may also be present. Physical examination often reveals tenderness to palpation in the lower lumbosacral spine and sacroiliac region. Lumbosacral movements may be painful and limited, especially forward flexion and extension. It is important to note that the presence or degree of lumbar degenerative spondylosis on imaging does not reliably correlate with the presence or severity of lumbosacral symptoms.

## LUMBOSACRAL RADICULOPATHY

Low back pain combined with neurogenic lower extremity pain (sciatica) strongly suggests lumbosacral nerve root irritation. Pain may be abrupt or gradual in onset, and it typically radiates from the buttock to the posterior or posterolateral thigh or to the ankle or foot. There may be accompanying lower-extremity numbness, tingling, or weakness. The knee-flexed position, either supine or side-lying, often affords relief. Physical examination is remarkable for abnormal posture (list to one side), variable lumbosacral tenderness and muscle spasm, and reduced lumbosacral ROM. Nerve stretch signs (e.g., SLR, femoral stretch sign) indicating lumbosacral root irritation are frequently present. Neurologic testing may indicate diminished reflexes, strength, or sensation in the affected root distribution. Almost 85% of lumbosacral disk herniations involve the L4/L5 (L5 nerve root) or L5/S1 (S1 nerve root) level. In most cases symptoms resolve without the need for surgery, although symptoms persist longer than typical mechanical low back pain.

Acute, severe low back pain with bilateral sciatica, saddle anesthesia, and recent-onset urinary dysfunction (retention, overflow incontinence) and/or loss of rectal sphincter tone strongly suggests a cauda equina syndrome.

## DEGENERATIVE LUMBAR SPINAL STENOSIS

Degenerative lumbar spinal stenosis is a relatively common cause of neurogenic lower-extremity pain in older individuals. Varying combinations of degenerative disk disease with loss of disk height, redundancy and hypertrophy of the ligamentum flavum, and occasionally degenerative spondylolisthesis lead to narrowing of the spinal canal with lateral recess or foraminal stenosis at multiple levels (Figure 8-15). Increased mechanical load on the facet joints combine with osteoarthritic changes and osteophyte formation. The onset of symptoms is typically insidious. The principal symptom is pain with tingling or numbness in one or both legs with standing, ambulation or spinal extension that is relieved by sitting or forward spinal flexion, but there may also be associated low back pain. Freedom from or improvement of symptoms during exercise in a flexed position (leaning on a grocery cart, walking uphill, bicycling) helps differentiate degenerative spinal stenosis from vascular claudication. Physical findings can include posterior thigh pain and transient motor weakness after 90 seconds of forced spinal extension, a wide-based gait, abnormal motor or sensory testing, and normal lower-extremity pulses. The physical examination is typically normal with the patient at rest, and the diagnosis is made primarily on the patient's history. Differential diagnosis includes hip disease, trochanteric bursitis, and peripheral neuropathy.

## WHIPLASH

It is important to understand that whiplash is only a mechanism of injury and not a description of any resulting structural damage. There is no clinical diagnosis of whiplash. The whiplash movement of the cervical spine most frequently occurs secondary to motor vehicle collisions or athletic injury. Acceleration and deceleration forces may result in injury to the intervertebral disks, apophyseal joints, and paraspinal soft tissues of the cervical spine. Patients may experience cervical discomfort with referral to shoulders or to the interscapular region, symptoms similar to mechanical neck pain. Neck symptoms without functional limitations are classified as Whiplash Associated Disorder I (WAD I); when there are associated functional limitations, as WAD II; as WAD III when radicular symptoms are present; and WAD IV when the injury results in cervical spine fracture or dislocation. Physical examination findings in WAD I and WAD II are similar to those found with mechanical neck pain, and typical findings in cervical radiculopathy have been described previously. When WAD IV is suspected, patients should be referred for appropriate orthopedic assessment.

## SPINAL FRACTURE

The evaluation of spinal pain immediately following major trauma, motor vehicle collisions, athletic injury, or worksite injury primarily involves the identification of fracture or dislocation. The clinical setting and initial screening history

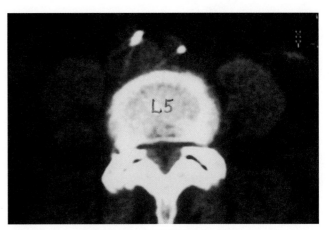

**FIGURE 8-15  AXIAL LUMBAR COMPUTED TOMOGRAPHIC SCAN: DEGENERATIVE SPINAL STENOSIS.** (Discovertebral degenerative changes, facet joint osteoarthritis, and ligamentum flavum hypertrophy).

should identify such patients, and an appropriate orthopedic assessment can be initiated.

Acute thoracic or lumbar spine pain associated with lesser trauma or injury—such as a minor fall, twisting, or heavy lifting in an older individual—raises the possibility of an osteoporotic fracture.

## THORACIC COMPRESSION FRACTURE

Osteoporotic compression fracture of a mid thoracic to lower thoracic vertebra is one of the common causes of acute thoracic spine pain in the elderly. Risk factors include advanced age, female sex, personal or family history of fracture, cigarette smoking, low body weight, estrogen or testosterone deficiency, and corticosteroid use. Acute, severe spine pain, especially when accompanied by radiation bilaterally around the rib cage, strongly suggests a compression fracture. Focal spinal tenderness to palpation or gentle percussion, in the absence of neurologic symptoms or signs of malignancy or infection, increases the likelihood of a possible compression fracture.

## INFLAMMATORY SPINAL PAIN

Spinal involvement in the spondyloarthropathies (e.g., ankylosing spondylitis, reactive arthritis, and spondylitis of inflammatory bowel disease) may involve the low back, thoracic spine, or neck and tends to occur early in the course of the disease. Initial symptoms are frequently vague and often overlooked. Characteristic features of inflammatory spondyloarthropathies include age less than 40 years, an insidious onset, significant morning stiffness, improvement of spinal pain with exercise and worsening with prolonged rest, awakening in the second half of the night with spinal pain, and a symptom duration of longer than 3 months. Although not specific, these features strongly suggest inflammatory back pain and are quite different from mechanical low back pain. The presence of SI joint pain and tenderness, limited spinal movements, and reduced chest expansion should prompt further investigation, most importantly an anteroposterior pelvic radiograph (Ferguson view) to check for radiographic sacroiliitis (Figure 8-16).

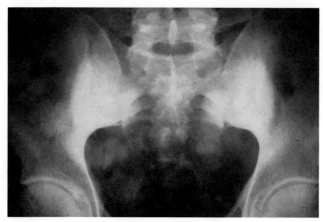

**FIGURE 8-16 ANTEROPOSTERIOR RADIOGRAPH OF THE PELVIS.** A 20° caudal tube angle showing bilateral sacroiliitis.

Spinal involvement in rheumatoid arthritis is confined to the neck and tends to occur late in the course of erosive disease. Inflammatory synovitis may cause progressive laxity of the ligaments between C1 and C2, resulting in atlantoaxial instability, and/or lower cervical intervertebral instability, resulting in subaxial subluxation. Despite the seriousness of these lesions, there may be little or no neck pain.

## SELECTED READINGS

Accident Compensation Corporation (ACC), 2004. New Zealand Acute Low Back Pain Guide. New Zealand, New Zealand Guidelines Group, Wellington.

Barnsley, L., 2003. Neck pain. In: Hochberg, M.C., Silman, A.J., Smolen, J.S. et al (Eds.), Rheumatology, third ed. Mosby, Edinburgh, UK, pp. 567–581.

Bigos, S.J., Bowyer, O.R., Braen, G.R., et al., 1994. Acute Low Back Problems in Adults. Clinical Practice Guidelines No. 14. Agency for Health Care Policy and Research, Public Health Service, US Dept. of Health and Health Services, Rockville, MD Publication No. 95-0642.

Carroll, L.J., Hogg-Johnson, S., van der Velde, G., et al., 2008. Course and prognostic factors for neck pain in the general population: results of the Bone and Joint Decade 2000-2010 Task Force on Neck Pain and Its Associated Disorders. Spine 33 (4 Suppl), S75–S82 Review.

Chou, R., Fu, R., Carrino, J.A., Deyo, R.A., 2009. Imaging strategies for low-back pain: systematic review and meta-analysis. Lancet 373 (9662), 463–472 Review.

Chou, R., Qaseem, A., Snow, V., et al., 2007. Clinical Efficacy Assessment Subcommittee of the American College of Physicians; American College of Physicians; American Pain Society Low Back Pain Guidelines Panel. Diagnosis and treatment of low back pain: a joint clinical practice guideline from the American College of Physicians and the American Pain Society. Ann. Intern. Med. 147 (7), 478–491.

Croft, P.R., Macfarlane, G.J., Papageorgiou, A.C., et al., 1998. Outcome of low back pain in general practice: a prospective study. Br. Med. J. 316 (7141), 1356–1359.

Dagenais, S., Caro, J., Haldeman, S., 2008. A systematic review of low back pain cost of illness studies in the United States and internationally. The Spine Journal 8 (1), 8–20.

Deyo, R.A., Diehl, A.K., 1988. Cancer as a Cause of Back Pain. J. Gen. Intern. Med. 3, 230–238.

Deyo, R.A., Weinstein, J.N., 2001. Low back pain. N. Engl. J. Med. 344, 363–370.

Deyo, R.A., 2002. Diagnostic evaluation of LBP: Reaching a specific diagnosis is often impossible. Arch. Intern. Med. 162, 1444–1447.

Guzmán, J., Esmail, R., Karjalainen, K., et al., 2001. Multidisciplinary rehabilitation for chronic low back pain: systematic review. Br. Med. J. 322 (7301), 1511–1516 Review.

Guzman, J., Haldeman, S., Carroll, L.J., et al., 2008. Bone and Joint Decade 2000-2010 Task Force on Neck Pain and Its Associated Disorders. Clinical practice implications of the Bone and Joint Decade 2000-2010 Task Force on Neck Pain and Its Associated Disorders: from concepts and findings to recommendations. Spine 33 (4 Suppl), S199–S213 Review.

Hall, H., McIntosh, G., Wilson, L., Melles, T., 1998. The spontaneous onset of back pain. Clin. J. Pain 14 (2), 129–133.

Hall, H., McIntosh, G., Boyle, C., 2009. Effectiveness of a low back pain classification system. The Spine Journal 9 (8), 648–657.

Hart, L.G., Deyo, R.A., Cherkin, D.C., 1995. Physician office visits for low back pain: Frequency, clinical evaluation and treatment patterns from a US national survey. Spine 20, 11–19.

Jarvik, J.G., Deyo, R.A., 2002. Diagnostic evaluation of low back pain with emphasis on imaging. Ann. Intern. Med. 137 (7), 586–597.

Katz, J.N., Harris, M.B., 2008. Clinical practice. Lumbar spinal stenosis. N. Engl. J. Med. 358 (8), 818–825 Review.

Kendrick, D., Fielding, K., Bentley, E., et al., 2001. The role of radiography in primary care patients with low back pain of at least 6 weeks duration: a randomised (unblinded) controlled trial. Health Technol Assess 5 (30), 1–69.

Kerry, S., Hilton, S., Dundas, D., et al., 2002. Radiography for low back pain: a randomised controlled trial and observational study in primary care. Br. J. Gen. Prac. 52 (479), 469–474.

Koes, B., van Tulder, M., Ostelo, R., et al., 2001. Clinical guidelines for the management of low back pain in primary care. Spine 26 (22), 2504–2514.

McCombe, P.F., Fairbank, J.C.T., Cockersole, B.C., et al., 1989. Reproducibility of physical signs in low back pain. Spine 14, 908–918.

Nordin, M., Carragee, E.J., Hogg-Johnson, S., et al., 2008. Bone and Joint Decade 2000-2010 Task Force on Neck Pain and Its Associated Disorders. Assessment of neck pain and its associated disorders: results of the Bone and Joint Decade 2000-2010 Task Force on Neck Pain and Its Associated Disorders. Spine 33 (4 Suppl), S101–S122 Review.

Suarez-Almazor, M.E., Belseck, E., Russell, A.S., Mackel, J.V., 1997. Use of Lumbar Radiographs for the Early Diagnosis of Low Back Pain. J. Am. Med. Assoc. 277 (22), 1782–1786.

van den Hoogen, H.J., Koes, B.W., van Eijk, J.T., et al., 1998. On the course of low back pain in general practice: a one-year follow up study. Ann. Rheum. Dis. 57 (1), 13–19.

Viikaru-Juntura, E., Porras, M., Laasonen, E.M., 1989. Validity of clinical tests in the diagnosis of root compression in cervical disc disease. Spine 14, 253–257.

Vroomen, P.C., deKrom, M.C., Knottnerus, J.A., 1999. Diagnostic value of history and physical examination in patients suspected of sciatica due to disc herniation: A systemic review. J. Neurol. 246, 899–906.

Waddell, G., McCullogh, J.A., Kummel, E., et al., 1980. Non-organic physical signs in low back pain. Spine 5, 117–125.

# 9

# THE TEMPOROMANDIBULAR JOINT

Michael B. Goldberg • Howard C. Tenenbaum • Bruce V. Freeman • Adel G. Fam

## Applied Anatomy

The temporomandibular joint (TMJ) is an articulation between the mandibular condyle and both the mandibular (glenoid) fossa and the articular eminence (tubercle) of the temporal bone (Figure 9-1). The paired TMJs are classified as **condylar joints,** because the mandible articulates with the skull by means of two distinct articular surfaces, or condyles. Unlike other synovial (diarthrodial) articulations, the articulating surfaces of the TMJ are covered by fibrocartilage in place of hyaline cartilage. An **intraarticular fibrocartilaginous disk (meniscus)** divides the joint into a large superior and a smaller inferior compartment, each lined with synovial membrane (see Figure 9-1). The disk consists of a thin, central portion; a thick, large, highly innervated and more vascular posterior portion (posterior band); and a smaller anterior portion (anterior band). The disk is tightly bound to the medial and lateral poles of the mandibular condyle. It provides congruent contours, acts as a shock absorber during mastication, and stabilizes the joint during mandibular movements. The stability of the TMJ depends on the osseous, conformation, muscles of mastication, capsule, ligaments, and intraarticular disk. The **capsule** is thin and loose and allows a wide range of movements. It is attached to the condyle and to the articular eminence, and it is reinforced on the lateral aspect by the **lateral temporomandibular ligament** and on the medial aspect by the **sphenomandibular ligament.**

### MOVEMENTS

Mastication, swallowing, and speech are associated with movements at the TMJs. The two joints move in unison and are limited and guided by dental occlusion during early opening and closing movements of the jaw. Therefore, the TMJs and teeth are often referred to as a *tri-joint complex.* However, later movements, beyond 2 mm opening, are guided by the musculoligamentous components of the TMJ and are not related to dental occlusion or bite. Movements at the TMJs have two components: *rotation,* which occurs during the very first stages of jaw opening, and *translation,* which occurs with wider opening. These movements are guided by the various components of the TMJ system and structure. The **inferior compartment** of the joint, between the mandibular condyle and the articular disk, functions as a hinge joint that allows mandibular rotation. The upper head of the lateral pterygoid muscle draws the disk anteriorly to prepare for condylar rotation. The **superior compartment** of the joint, between the temporal bone and the articular disk, acts as a sliding joint; it allows both disk and mandible to glide anteriorly, posteriorly, and laterally (left or right) along the slope of the articular eminence. The eminence is the primary functional area of the temporal bone during mandibular movement. Normal opening and closing of the mouth, a combination of rotation and translation movements, relies on function in both compartments of each joint. Further, it depends on a smooth sliding of the disk down the slope of the eminence. During mouth opening, the condyles glide forward over the articular eminence with the disk in between. Therefore, during mouth opening, the condyles rest on the articular eminences, and any sudden movement, such as wide mouth opening that might occur during yawning, and some forms of trauma may displace one or both condyles anteriorly and even past the articular eminence, a process that can lead to open lock of the mandible.

In the closed position, the mandible lies in the glenoid fossa, in contact with the posterior band of the disk (see Figure 9-1). In the **resting position,** the mouth is slightly open so that the teeth are not in contact. In **centric occlusion** occurs with maximal contact of the teeth, the position assumed by the jaw when swallowing.

### TEETH

In humans, there are 20 deciduous—primary or "baby"—teeth, and 32 secondary, or permanent, teeth. Deciduous teeth are shed between the ages of 6 and 13 years. To identify or label the secondary teeth for the purposes of communication and treatment, their locations are divided into four quadrants: *upper left* (quadrant 1), *upper right* (quadrant 2), *lower left* (quadrant 3), and *lower right* (quadrant 4). When labeling or identifying deciduous teeth, the quadrants are continued so that deciduous teeth would be found in quadrants 5 through 8, with quadrant 5 being the deciduous "partner" of quadrant 1, used for secondary teeth and so on. In each quadrant, the teeth are numbered from 1 (most medial) to 8 (most distal). Therefore, a mandibular right first molar would be called tooth 4.6, or simply 46, and a first mandibular deciduous molar on the right side would be labeled tooth 8.5, or 85. Loss or restoration of teeth and malocclusion has been considered a major factor in the development of TMJ pain. Although this used to be considered a major risk factor for TMJ dysfunction, unless the occlusal changes are so great as to render the occlusion nonfunctional (e.g., no posterior

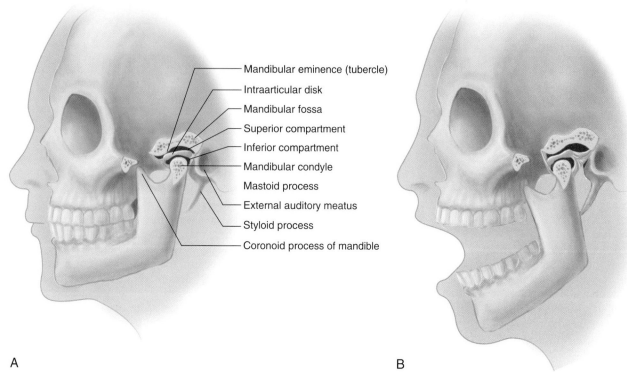

Mandibular eminence (tubercle)
Intraarticular disk
Mandibular fossa
Superior compartment
Inferior compartment
Mandibular condyle
Mastoid process
External auditory meatus
Styloid process
Coronoid process of mandible

A                                                                                   B

**FIGURE 9-1   THE TEMPOROMANDIBULAR JOINT. A,** Mouth closed: Mandibular condyle and disk lie within the mandibular fossa.
**B,** Mouth open: The mandibular condyle and disk glide forward and lie over the articular eminence.

occlusion at all), it is no longer considered as such (De Boever, 2000).

## NERVE SUPPLY

The TMJs are innervated by the auriculotemporal and masseteric branches of the mandibular division of the trigeminal nerve.

## Temporomandibular Joint Pain and History Taking

Pain reported in the TMJ is a relatively common symptom, but it can have diverse causes. It may originate in the TMJ itself, or it may be referred from the teeth, ear, parotid gland, muscles of mastication, cervical spine, or head (Table 9-1). Important points in the history include site, duration, character, radiation, and provocative factors of TMJ pain. The physician may also inquire about any recent dental work and whether a patient grinds the teeth. Both **bruxism**—forced clenching and grinding of the teeth, especially during sleep— and **habitual nail biting** have been associated with a temporomandibular disorder syndrome, which will be discussed later. However, these are basically associations and to date have not been demonstrated to be causal. That said, these characteristics might have an impact on pain severity, timing, and responsiveness to treatment. In fact, apart from TMJ pain syndromes that arise following hyperextension-flexion injury, most of these conditions are idiopathic in nature (Romanelli, 1992; Goldberg, 1996; and Brooke, 1978).

**Locking** of the TMJs can be caused by subluxation of the joint or, more likely, may be caused by anterior displacement without reduction of the meniscus (i.e., TMJ disk). **Clicking, popping, or snapping** of TMJs, often bilateral, occurs when the TMJ disk is positioned anterior to its normal position. However, in contrast to a locked joint, opening movement that requires translation of the TMJs can cause popping or clicking in one or both of these joints that may be audible or at least detected by palpation. This phenomenon occurs because the joint actually snaps back over the displaced disk, leading to the reestablishment of a normal relationship between the condyle and the central zone of the disk (Westesson, 1985). Other causes of clicking and popping can include a meniscal tear, uncoordinated lateral pterygoid muscle action, and osteoarthritis (OA).

## Physical Examination

### INSPECTION

The TMJs are inspected for pain, swelling, redness, symmetry, clicking, crepitus, abnormal movements such as asymmetric translation, lack of movement, and hypermobility. Effusion of the TMJ manifests as a rounded bulge just anterior to the external auditory meatus. Arthritis of the TMJs, particularly rheumatoid (and not OA), can predispose to the development of an obvious anterior open bite, in which the patient cannot bring his or her anterior teeth together (e.g., to bite off a piece of thread). In children this might also result in the development of a disturbance of bone growth leading to a shortened, recessed lower jaw

## TABLE 9-1

### DIFFERENTIAL DIAGNOSIS OF TEMPOROMANDIBULAR JOINT (TMJ) PAIN

**Arthritis of the TMJ**

Osteoarthritis (OA)
Rheumatoid arthritis (RA)
Psoriatic arthritis (PsA)
Ankylosing spondylitis (AS)
Juvenile idiopathic arthritis (JIA)
Trauma
Infection
Gout

**Temporomandibular Disorder Syndrome (TMDS)**

**Internal Derangement due to Meniscal Displacement**

**Condylar Agenesis, Hypoplasia (Retrognathism), and Hyperplasia (Prognathism)**

**Neoplasms of the TMJ (rare)**

Chondroma
Osteochondroma
Osteoma

**Referred TMJ Pain**

From the parotid salivary gland
From the paranasal sinuses
From the ear
From the teeth
From the nasopharynx
From the cervical spine

**Other Causes of Facial Pain**

Trigeminal neuralgia
Giant cell (temporal) arteritis
Migraine headache
Cerebral tumors, tetanus, Parkinsonism
Fibromyalgia
Psychosomatic TMJ pain

and excessive overjet. While excessive overjet may result from various causes, be they congenital or acquired, there are no studies revealing a conclusive relationship between factors of occlusion, such as overjet and overbite, with the development of temporomandibular dysfunction (TMD) (Gersh et al, 2004). It should also be recognized that other diseases can cause lysis or destruction of one or both TMJs, including neoplasia (benign or malignant), and these must be ruled out in the absence of a history consistent with adult or juvenile rheumatoid disease.

## PALPATION

The TMJs can be located by placing the tip of the index finger just anterior to the external auditory meatus and asking the patient to open the mouth about halfway. The lateral poles of the TMJs will then become palpable by the tip of the examiner's finger. The joint is palpated for warmth, tenderness, synovial thickening, effusion (a fluctuant mass), crepitus, or snapping or clicking with movement. With the patient's mouth open, the TMJ can be palpated with the little finger placed in the external auditory meatus (fleshy part anteriorly). The patient is then asked to close the mouth when the examiner first feels the condyle touch the finger. With the mouth closed, the TMJs are in the resting position with a

freeway space between the anterior teeth (normal range 2 to 4 mm) (Kerr, 1974). By palpating the condyle and noting its location within the mandibular fossa with the patient's mouth closed, partially open, and wide open, the examiner can determine various degrees of dislocation.

When assessing for pain, one generally tries to maintain a consistent force of palpation. If tissues are clinically tender, it is generally recommended that the force needed to evoke a meaningful pain reaction is that which, when pressing the finger on a tabletop, the fingernail bed will blanch. If the pressure is too light, clinically tender tissues will not be identified; similarly, if too much force is applied, even normal tissues will be perceived as painful. For the purposes of standardization, it is also helpful to grade a patient's pain reaction following palpation of the TMJs and surrounding musculature. In this case, a discontinuous but relatively reliable scale has been developed, as shown in Table 9-2.

## RANGE OF MOVEMENT

Active TMJ movements include opening and closing of the mouth, protrusion, retrusion, and lateral or side-to-side excursions of the mandible. During opening (depression) and closing (elevation or occlusion) of the mouth, the two TMJs (inferior compartments) work in unison to produce a smooth, unbroken arc of movement without any asymmetry or sideways movement. Deviation of the chin to one side is generally caused by ipsilateral TMJ, severe degenerative changes that would generally be seen only in rheumatoid arthritis, physical trauma (e.g., fracture of the neck of the ipsilateral condyle), and, in some cases, spasm of the masseter or lateral or medial pterygoid muscles.

The range of vertical movement during opening and closing of the mouth is determined by measuring, with a ruler or calipers, the **distance between** the maxillary and mandibular central incisors during maximal unassisted or assisted opening (see the discussion that follows on passive movements of the TMJ). This range is often referred to as the **interincisal range of opening** (normal range 35 to 60 mm). Although this measurement is relatively reproducible, inaccurate measurements can be made in patients wearing dentures or in those who have otherwise lost maxillary anterior teeth that have then been replaced prosthetically. In hypomobile TMJs, the distance is less than 35 mm, and the displacement can be so severe as to be less than or equal to 1.5 cm, therefore only rotational movement of the condyles would be detected.

Protrusion and retrusion of the mandible occur at the superior compartment. Normally, the individual can both protrude the lower jaw out past the upper teeth and retract the lower teeth behind the upper teeth. Lateral or side-to-side movement of the mandible occurs at the superior compartment. This can be measured with a ruler, with the mouth partially open and the lower jaw protruded, as the range of movement of the midpoint of the mandible (i.e., the space between two central incisors) in relation to that of the maxilla (normal range 10 to 20 mm).

As alluded to earlier, jaw opening can be characterized as being assisted or unassisted. Unassisted opening is generally close to assisted opening in extent, when there is no pain or other disease associated with either the TMJs or their

TABLE 9-2

## PAIN REACTIONS FOLLOWING PALPATION/EXAMINATION

| Grade 0 | Grade 1 | Grade 2 | Grade 3 |
|---------|---------|---------|---------|
| No pain reaction at all | Pain reaction not visible, but when asked, patient confirms pain | Visible pain reaction (movement, pupillary reaction) to palpation; patient does not have to be asked if there is pain | Visible pain reaction, often with marked avoidance on the part of the patient as well as audible reaction (That hurts!); might note grade 2–like reaction even before normal palpation force has been achieved |

When using this scale for the purpose of research studies, the first two categories are often concatenated and considered negative pain reactions, and grades 2 and 3 are concatenated and considered positive. This permits two-by-two analyses to be done and helps to reduce the effects of intraexaminer and interexaminer variability on outcomes. Finally, an extremely important diagnostic feature of palpation, particularly when considering diagnosis of pain, is whether or not the patient's chief pain complaint has been exacerbated following this type of examination. If not, the patient's primary pain might be related to another condition or to pain in other structures (e.g., the muscles that can be palpated separately). However, if the patient's primary pain *is* exacerbated following TMJ palpation, then the patient's pain is likely emanating from one or both TMJs.

associated muscles, and it is measured by having the patient open his or her mouth to its widest extent or to the point where pain interferes with such movement. Assisted opening is measured, with the examiner wearing gloves, by placing the middle finger on the incisal edges of either the maxillary or mandibular teeth and the thumb on the incisal edges of the opposing incisors. The thumb and middle finger are then brought together gently and slowly, in a scissors movement, to determine whether it is possible to assist the mandible to open more than it did with unassisted opening. In these cases, there might be too much pain to even do this. However, in most cases this maneuver can still be done. Presuming no intraarticular disease, such as an anteriorly displaced TMJ meniscus without reduction, and as long as there is no extremely severe pain, the mandible can be coaxed to open, sometimes another 1 to 2 cm. This is also parallel to the concept of a springy feeling at maximal opening and would generally be consistent with a diagnosis of muscular pain and/or muscle trismus that is causing a restriction in unassisted opening. Alternatively, if the mandible can only be coaxed to open another 1 to 5 cm, a so-called hard feeling will be detected. The latter finding often suggests intraarticular disease, such as an anteriorly displaced TMJ disk without reduction. Another condition that could cause this type of finding might be TMJ ankylosis related to trauma or other bone/joint disease, including infection, and it may require surgical intervention (Straith, 1948). Conditions associated with TMJ disk position and shape will be discussed in more detail later (see Temporomandibular Joint Pain and History Taking).

## MUSCLE TESTING AND NEUROLOGICAL ASSESSMENT

Although there is no question that patients will present with jaw-associated pain because of TMJ disease, it must also be recognized that pain in the surrounding muscles can also cause pain; in most instances, this is in fact the case (Dworkin, 1990). Moreover, most patients present with *both* muscular and TMJ pain. In cases of combined joint and muscle pain, the overall symptom profile and responses to treatment suggest that it is the muscular pain that is of paramount importance as opposed to pain strictly in the TMJ (Hapak, 1994). Therefore in addition to assessment of the TMJ itself, it is critically important to also test for muscle pain. Furthermore,

orofacial pain can arise as a consequence of dentoalveolar disease or neuropathy, which underscores the importance of carrying out an appropriate neurological assessment as well.

For neurological assessment, the patient is asked to close the jaws tightly for assessment of size, firmness, and strength of the temporalis and masseter muscles. Resisted isometric testing of the muscles that close the mouth is then performed, including the temporalis (innervated by facial or cranial nerve VII), the masseter (trigeminal or cranial nerve V), and the medial pterygoid (trigeminal nerve). This is followed by assessment of the muscles that open the mouth: the lateral pterygoid (trigeminal nerve) and the suprahyoid muscles—digastric (cranial nerves V and VII), mylohyoid (cranial nerve V), and geniohyoid (cranial nerve XII and the first cervical nerve, C1). Side-to-side movements of the mandible are a function of the medial and lateral pterygoids. Protrusion of the mandible is a function of the lateral pterygoids, whereas retrusion is produced by the posterior fibers of the temporalis. In patients with hypocalcemic tetany, tapping of the facial nerve, as it runs just in front of the tragus, produces a momentary spasm of the ipsilateral half of the face (positive **Chvostek test**). The **jaw reflex** is mediated by the trigeminal nerve.

When testing for pain in the muscles of mastication, it is important to examine the external muscles—masseter, temporalis, medial pterygoid at the angle of the mandible, and sternocleidomastoid—by palpation. The internal muscles must also be palpated; these include the masseter at its zygomatic attachment and the coronoid attachment of the temporalis. One can also palpate the medial pterygoid muscles, but this can also induce gagging, which makes it difficult to assess for pain reactions. The lateral pterygoid muscles are also palpated, but in reality, it is doubtful that they can actually be reached during a physical examination. The same amount of digital pressure on the muscles of mastication as described for palpation of the TMJs should be used. Similarly, the patient's pain reactions can be gauged using the measurement system described in Table 9-2. Equally as important, as discussed with respect to examination of the TMJs, a patient might or might not feel pain following palpation; if the patient *does* feel pain, *and* the patient's chief pain complaint has been exacerbated following palpation of the muscles of mastication, it can be concluded that the principal source of pain is muscular. That said, patients suffering from chronic muscle pain syndromes such as fibromyalgia, which is a common comorbid condition for patients with TMJ or associated pain in the muscles of mastication (Dao, 1997), might report severe pain following palpation; but their chief pain complaints might not be exacerbated. This latter type of finding should suggest a diagnosis of fibromyalgia, which would need further medical assessment, such as examination by a rheumatologist, neurologist, or physiatrist—three appropriate medical subspecialties concerned with these conditions.

## Common Musculoskeletal Disorders of the TMJ

### TEMPOROMANDIBULAR ARTHRITIS

**Temporomandibular (TM) arthritis** can be caused by trauma, infection, OA, rheumatoid arthritis (RA), psoriatic arthritis (PsA), ankylosing spondylitis (AS), juvenile idiopathic (rheumatoid) arthritis (JIA), or crystal-induced arthritis—such as gout, and even pseudogout—or calcium pyrophosphate dihydrate deposition arthropathy (Pritzker, 1994). In some rare cases, TM arthritis may be caused by malignant metastatic or primary disease. The pain of TM arthritis may radiate to the teeth, face, or ear, and it is made worse by jaw movements during eating, chewing, and speaking. With regard to OA, pain usually occurs once there is loss of the fibrous articular joint surface. As a result, the loss of this protective layer exposes the innervated and vascularized osseous tissue to the effects of movement and forces that result in pain (Okeson, 2005). Rheumatoid arthritides (including JIA) occur as a result of proliferation of inflamed synovial membranes onto the articular surfaces (Okeson, 2005). Other symptoms include stiffness, restriction of movement with inability to fully open the mouth, swelling, clicking, and sometimes locking. Local tenderness, swelling, synovial thickening, effusion, fine or coarse crepitus, and sometimes a palpable click are the main findings. In chronic arthritis, excessive play of the TMJ is common.

### TEMPOROMANDIBULAR DISORDER SYNDROME

Temporomandibular disorder syndrome (TMDS) is currently referred to as **temporomandibular disorder (TMD)** in recognition of the fact that this condition can be caused by TMJ pain and muscle pain, as well as combined TMJ and muscle pain as described previously. When the condition is predominantly caused by pain in the muscles of mastication, it can also be referred to as **myofascial pain** and **dysfunction (MPD)**. The first descriptions of this condition were made by Costen in 1934. TMD is a relatively frequent cause of chronic head and neck pain associated with dysfunction of the masticatory muscles. The pain is dull, achy in character, rarely relieved by analgesics, and when associated primarily with the muscles of mastication, is fairly diffuse. This is in contrast to TMJ-associated pain from one of the arthritides mentioned previously, in which the pain is typically localized to the joint area (i.e., just anterior to the external auditory meatus, also often mistaken for otitis media). The pain of TMD related to joint disease is often unilateral and is aggravated by jaw movements, but it is independent of any local oral, nasal, dental, or ear disease. Tenderness of the muscles of mastication can be identified, too; but if the condition is related mainly to joint disease, palpation of the joints, not the muscles, would be expected to exacerbate the patient's chief pain complaints.

### INTERNAL DERANGEMENTS

The disk displacements discussed previously are also referred to as **internal derangements.** The etiology is not understood fully, but impaired lubrication due to TMJ overloading has been implicated. Known causes include direct or indirect trauma (blow to the jaw, endotracheal intubation), abnormal functional loading of the joint (bruxism, chronic teeth clenching), and OA. It is noteworthy that internal derangement is so common that it has been suggested that, unless associated with pain or severely restricted opening, it is more a variation of normal as opposed to true disease.

Clinically, there is a painless incoordination phase initially, during which the patient experiences a momentary catching sensation on mouth opening. This is followed by the clicking and popping associated with anterior disk displacement and reduction into the normal position with mouth opening. Some patients may subsequently develop restricted jaw movements with intermittent or permanent locking caused by anterior disk displacement without reduction on attempted mouth opening. The common factor here is that in such cases, almost all patients would have reported prior TMJ noises with jaw opening and/or closing (a reciprocal click) prior to the development of closed lock. Furthermore, on development of a closed lock caused by anterior displacement without reduction, the patient will also report that the clicking is no longer present. The diagnosis of internal derangement can be confirmed by magnetic resonance imaging (MRI); but in fact, history and clinical examination are just as sensitive (Romanelli et al, 1993).

## Management

Although abnormal TMJ signs, mostly joint noises or clicking, are relatively common, symptoms are less frequent, and only a minority of patients seek medical advice for them. Treatment of painless TMJ clicking is not recommended, unless the condition is seriously bothering the patient. If the clicking is painful, treatment is indicated and can include treatment with an intraoral appliance known as *a biteplane.* Some clinicians advocate for a biteplane that positions the mandible anteriorly so as to "recapture" the disk (Gelb, 1979). In some cases arthroscopic surgery is performed, also to recapture and/or repair the disk, and this might be aided by viscosupplementation, placement of hyaluronate into the TMJ capsule following arthroscopic surgery. Alternatively, a procedure called **arthrocentesis** has also been shown to be effective in either reducing the symptoms of clicking or at least reducing the associated pain. In fact, arthrocentesis is a component of arthroscopic surgery, which will be discussed in more detail later, and could actually be the most important part of the treatment that leads to improvement (Tenenbaum, 1999). The goals of arthrocentesis are not to recapture or repair the joint but to lavage inflammatory byproducts out of the joint capsule and to then replace the joint fluid with hyaluronate and/or a corticosteroid. Interestingly, most evidence suggests that in spite of treatment, displaced TMJ menisci are not recaptured and do not return to a normal position—and yet patients still report clinically significant improvement in their pain symptoms, if not the clicking (Nitzan, 1991 and Freeman, 1997). Another useful, noninvasive treatment modality is physiotherapy that involves manipulation, massage, moist heat, and jaw exercises (Rocabado, 1982).

## LOCAL ASPIRATION AND INJECTION/ ARTHROSCOPIC TREATMENTS

When considering treatment of an inflamed TMJ, local aspiration and injection of the joint may be required, with a steroid and/or with hyaluronate. With the patient sitting or reclining and the head supported, the joint line is palpated as a depression located 1 to 2 cm anterior to the tragus, and the mandibular condyle is felt as it moves during mouth opening and closing. With the patient's mouth open, a 27 gauge needle is inserted into the joint perpendicular to the skin and directed slightly posteriorly, medially, and superiorly, with care being taken not to inject directly into the intraarticular disk (Figure 9-2). The ease of injection and/or aspiration of fluid is the best guide to ensure that the needle's point is within the joint cavity. Generally speaking, local anesthesia should be established as per routine when carrying out such procedures. More recent developments in this approach, and with arthrocentesis in particular, require a similar approach but also involve the development of a draining channel with a second needle. This allows for inflammatory cytokines (e.g., prostaglandins) to be flushed from the joint capsule, followed by placement of the steroid and/or hyaluronate. It should be noted that if a patient's pain is *not* alleviated following local anesthetic administration into the joint,

presuming the patient is in pain at the time of presentation, the patient's pain is likely not emanating from the joint. This would mean that another source of pain should be considered; as alluded to earlier, this is likely to be muscular, presuming other sources of pain, such as dentoalveolar pain and otitis media, have been eliminated diagnostically. Therefore, injection of the TMJ is not only a possible therapeutic measure, it can be used for diagnostic purposes as well.

Arthroscopic methods can be used to guide aspiration and injection along with surgical management of intraarticular disease. Interestingly, studies focused on the use of arthroscopic surgery have shown that surgical outcomes can be affected by the presence and/or severity of a psychopathological disorder (Freeman, 1997; Dworkin, 1994; and Murray, 1996). The various investigations have demonstrated that the biomechanical aspects of jaw function—as measured directly and objectively, as with maximal mandibular opening (MMO)—were unaltered following arthroscopic surgery. In parallel, the incidence and severity of TMJ sounds did not change following surgical treatment. However, there were marked reductions in pain (> 60%). Moreover, although there were no changes in the objective measurements of either MMO or joint noises, based on measurements made with visual analog scales, patients perceived at least 60% reductions in joint noises that also correlated with similar perceptions in their maximal jaw opening. These data suggest that although biomechanical function might be an important parameter insofar as joint function is concerned, pain might be the overriding symptom; when pain is reduced, patients seem to perceive that their biomechanical problems (i.e., maximal jaw opening) have improved to a similar extent.

## INJECTION OF MUSCLES OF MASTICATION

When it is suspected that a patient's symptoms are related to painful muscles of mastication, diagnostic, and in some cases therapeutic, injection of local anesthetics may be considered with or without a corticosteroid. As suggested for injection of the TMJ, the administration of a local anesthetic prior to placement of a steroid, if a steroid is to be used, should also lead to elimination or at least reduction in the patient's chief pain complaints. These injections can be therapeutic (Wheeler, 2004) or at least diagnostic. Both internal and external muscles of mastication can be injected, depending on what muscles were shown to be tender to palpation; in general it is suggested that when the muscles are injected with a local anesthetic, it should be done without a vasoconstrictor. Dry needling has also been used, but its effectiveness is questionable (Furlan et al, 2003).

## PREDICTION OF TREATMENT OUTCOMES FOR TMD AND ASSOCIATED MUSCULOLIGAMENTOUS PAIN CONDITIONS

Predicting treatment outcome in chronic pain cases, and with temporomandibular disorders in particular, is one of the most challenging aspects of managing these conditions. Unlike more conventional medical and dental models, in which the response to treatment is based on a number of well-defined interventions, chronic pain management provides numerous challenges not observed in other conditions. The biopsychosocial model used to explain the etiology of

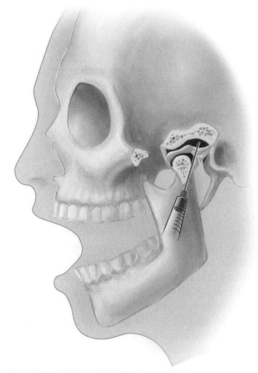

**FIGURE 9-2** ARTHROCENTESIS OF THE TEMPOROMANDIBULAR JOINT.

chronic pain may provide some insight into the variability of patient outcomes. Additionally, the originating trigger to the complaint, such as a motor vehicle accident, and other cofactors, including sleep disturbance and fibromyalgia, have been shown to play a significant role in determining the outcome of therapy.

In general, patients presenting with idiopathic TMD (iTMD)—those conditions not associated with a traumatic origin—recover in approximately 75% to 80% of cases (Brooke, 1977). Contrary to this observation, those patients presenting with signs and symptoms associated with a temporomandibular disorder with an onset in conjunction with a motor vehicle accident (pTMD) tend to do poorly in treatment and require more modalities of therapy than those patients that do improve. In fact, only about 48% of post-traumatic temporomandibular disorder sufferers suggest that they improved following conservative therapy (Romanelli, 1992). It has been suggested that those suffering from signs and symptoms associated with pTMD demonstrate a greater incidence of sleep disturbance, decreased energy level, mood swings, problems with cognitive functioning, and memory and concentration disturbances. These characteristics are similar to those seen in patients suffering from post-traumatic stress disorder (PTSD) (Afari, 2008). Yet in most TMD populations, there is no overt neurological deficit identified. Thus, it has been suggested that further characterization of these conditions, in particular those temporomandibular disorders that are more refractory to treatment, via the use of neuropsychological testing similar to that used in the post-traumatic TMD group may be helpful in not only assessing common features but may assist in formulating a more accurate diagnosis early in therapy.

A number of neuropsychological tests are available for assessment of cognitive functioning. However, some of the more common tests include a simple and complex reaction-time test, the California Verbal Learning Test, the Peterson-Peterson Consonant Trigram Test, and the Symptom Checklist-90 revised (SCL 90R). It has been suggested that individuals who have suffered from a head injury may develop difficulties with information processing. Therefore, the reaction-time tests and memory tests that assess the ability to encode information, including short and long-term memory function, may all be reflective of a cognitive deficit despite a normal neurological examination. It has been demonstrated by Goldberg et al (1996). that patients presenting with TMD symptoms associated with a motor vehicle accident did worse on reaction time and cognitive function tests compared to those suffering from a TMD of an idiopathic origin.

Following up on this work, it was suggested that neuropsychological deficits may play an integral role in mediating poor treatment outcomes in TMD patients. Accordingly, using various neuropsychological testing tools, as was done in the pTMD population, may provide some form of predictor in terms of poor treatment outcomes in the iTMD population. Although reaction-time testing was shown to be a poor predictor of treatment outcomes, other neuropsychological parameters described in the California Verbal Learning Test and the Peterson-Peterson Consonant Trigram Test were able to discriminate between responders and nonresponders in an iTMD population (Grossi, 2001). Conceivably, these tests might be utilized to predict poor outcomes

and thereby funnel patients into therapies to improve memory and cognition, which may in turn improve outcomes overall. Similarly, it has been demonstrated that these findings may be extrapolated to other chronic pain conditions, such as irritable bowel syndrome, with consistent findings noted (Grossi, 2008).

One of the overriding factors associated with chronic pain, and with TMD in particular, is the presence of a sleep disturbance. Chronic diffuse myalgia, fibromyalgia, and chronic fatigue syndrome are just some of the conditions associated with chronic sleep disturbance (Moldofsky, 1993). Along with that, it has been demonstrated that post-traumatic TMD patients are more likely to claim to suffer from a sleep disturbance and other symptoms related to affect than a comparative nontraumatic TMD population (60% vs. 14%) (Romanelli, 1992). However, in those that are considered refractory to treatment, it was demonstrated that on average, the nonresponding TMD population performed worse on most cognitive tests than those TMD patients who responded to treatment. Additionally, results of the University of Toronto Sleep Assessment Questionnaire (SAQ) indicated that elements of a sleep disturbance may have been present in the nonresponsive TMD group, although the diagnosis of a sleep disturbance could not be definitively made (Grossi, 2001). Overall, however, studies on TMD and sleep disturbance are limited. It has been reported that as many as 77% of those suffering from orofacial pain suffer from a sleep disturbance (Riley, 2001). The sleep–pain relationship is complicated by mood (Menefee et al, 2000), with poor sleepers endorsing higher scores on measures of depression and anxiety (Haythornthwaite, 1991). In a sample of patients with orofacial pain, sleep quality was predicted by depressed mood or psychological distress and greater pain severity and less perceived life control (Yatani et al, 2002). However, in a study assessing psychological and cognitive variables that may be predictive of positive outcomes in TMD patients undergoing physiotherapy treatment, it was determined that neuropsychological test results, as well as sleep quality, were not able to predict treatment outcome in any meaningful way (Bielawski, 2008). Although many factors may contribute to the etiology and pathogenesis of TMDs, it is still beyond our ability to accurately predict those who will or will not respond to therapy, no matter which modality is utilized.

## Conclusions

Clearly, factors that affect chronic pain in other joints and associated musculature within the body play an equally important role with regard to problems surrounding the TMJ and the muscles of mastication. What makes this structural complex so different is that pain in and around the TMJ and its muscles can arise from several sources, ranging from dentoalveolar to muscular origins. Moreover, it is also clear from findings now reported in the literature, and as described in this final section, that higher-center control of pain and suffering (i.e., the central nervous system) plays an extremely important role in relation to chronicity of pain regardless of the anatomical location of the pain. Mounting data suggest that apart from clearly biomechanical problems associated with joint movements, and indeed even when biomechanical problems seem to explain any one patient's symptoms, manipulation of pain perception, possibly with the use of treatment approaches that rely more heavily on cognitive behavioral therapy (CBT) (Flor, 1993), might prove to be as useful, if not more so, in management of joint-associated pain than some surgical or more invasive treatment methods currently in use.

## REFERENCES

Afari, N., Wen, Y., Buchwald, D., et al., 2008. Are post-traumatic stress disorder symptoms and temporomandibular pain associated? Findings from a community-based twin registry. J. Orofacial Pain 22 (1), 41–49.

Bielawski, D.M., 2008. Treatment Response to Physical Therapy in Patients with Temporomandibular Disorders. Master's Thesis, Faculty of Dentistry, University of Toronto.

Brooke, R.I., Stenn, P.G., 1978. Postinjury myofascial pain dysfunction syndrome: Its etiology and prognosis. Oral Surg. 45, 846–850.

Brooke, R.I., Stenn, P.G., Mothersill, K.J., 1977. The diagnosis and conservative treatment of myofascial pain dysfunction syndrome. Oral Surg. Oral Med. Oral Pathol. 44 (6), 844–852.

Dao, T.T., Reynolds, W.J., Tenenbaum, H.C., 1997. Comorbidity between myofascial pain of the masticatory muscles and fibromyalgia. J. Orofacial Pain 11 (3), 232–241.

De Boever, J.A., Carlsson, G.E., Klineberg, I.J., 2000. Need for occlusal therapy and prosthodontic treatment in the management of temporomandibular disorders. Part II: tooth loss and prosthodontic treatment. J. Oral Rehab. 27 (8), 647–659.

Dworkin, S.F., Huggins, K.H., LeResch, L., et al., 1990. Epidemiology of signs and symptoms in temporomandibular disorders: Clinical signs in cases and controls. J. Am. Dent. Assoc. 120, 273–281.

Dworkin, S.F., Massoth, D.L., 1994. Temporomandibular Disorders And Chronic Pain: Disease Or Illness? J. Prosthetic Dentistry 72, 29–38.

Flor, H., Birbaumer, N., 1993. Comparison of the Efficacy of Electromyographic Biofeedback, Cognitive-Behavioral Therapy, and Conservative Medical Interventions in the Treatment of Chronic Musculoskeletal Pain. J. Consult. Clin. Psychol. 61 (4), 653–658.

Freeman, B.V., 1997. The Effect of Psychopathological Disorders on the Outcome of Temporomandibular Joint Arthroscopic Surgery: A Comparison of Objective and Subjective Outcome Measures. Master's Thesis, Faculty of Dentistry, University of Toronto, p. 52.

Furlan, A.D., van Tulder, M.W., Cherkin, D., et al., 2003. Acupuncture and dry needling for low back pain. Cochrane Database of Systematic Reviews (Issue 2).

Gelb, H., 1979. An orthopedic approach to occlusal imbalance and temporomandibular joint dysfunction. Dental Clin. Nor. Am. 23 (2), 181–197.

Gersh, D., Bernhardt, O., 2004. Angle Orthodontist 74 (4), 512–520.

Goldberg, M.B., Mock, D., Ichise, M., et al., 1996. Neuropsychologic Deficits and Clinical Features of Posttraumatic Temporomandibular Disorders. J. Orofacial Pain 10, 126–140.

Grossi, M.L., Goldberg, M.B., Locker, D., Tenenbaum, H.C., 2001. Reduced Neuropsychologic Measures as Predictors of Treatment Outcome in Patients with Temporomandibular Disorders. J. Orofacial Pain 15, 329–339.

Grossi, M.L., Goldberg, M.B., Locker, D., Tenenbaum, H.C., 2008. Irritable Bowel Syndrome Patients Versus Responding and nonresponding Temporomandibular Disorder Patients: A Neuropsychologic Profile Comparative Study. Int. J. Prosthodont 21, 201–209.

Hapak, L., Gordon, A., Locker, D., et al., 1994. Differentiation between musculoligamentous, dentoalveolar, and neurologically based craniofacial pain with a diagnostic questionnaire. J. Orofacial Pain 8 (4), 357–368.

Haythornthwaite, J.A., Sieber, W.J., Kerns, R.D., 1991. Depression and the chronic pain experience. Pain 46, 177–184.

Kerr, D.A., Ahs, M.M., Millard, H.D., 1974. Oral Diagnosis, fourth ed. Mosby, St. Louis.

Menefee, L.A., Frank, E.D., Doghramji, K., et al., 2000. Self-reported Sleep Quality and Quality of Life for Individuals with Chronic Pain Conditions. Clin. J Pain 16 (4), 290–297.

Moldofsky, H., 1993. Fibromyalgia, sleep disorder and chronic fatigue syndrome. Ciba Found. Symp. 173, 262–271.

Murray, H., Locker, D., Mock, D., Tenenbaum, H.C., 1996. Pain And The Quality Of Life In Patients Referred To A Craniofacial Pain Unit. J. Orofacial Pain 10, 316–323.

Nitzan, D.W., Dolwick, M.F., Martinez, A., 1991. Temporomandibular Joint Arthrocentesis: A Simplified Treatment for Severe, Limited Mouth Opening. J. Oral Maxillofac. Surg. 49 (11), 1163–1167.

Okeson, J.P. (Ed.), 2005. Bell's Orofacial Pains: the Clinical Management of Orofacial Pain. In Quintessence, sixth ed, p. 329, 353.

Pritzker, K.P., 1994. Calcium pyrophosphate dihydrate crystal deposition and other crystal deposition diseases. Curr. Opin. Rheum. 6 (4), 442–447.

Riley, J.L., Benson, M.B., Gremillion, H.A., et al., 2001. Sleep disturbance in orofacial pain patients: pain-related or emotional distress? Cranio. 19 (2), 106–113.

Rocabado, M., Johnston Jr., B.E., Blakney, M.G., 1982. Physical Therapy and Dentistry: An Overview. J. Craniomandibular Pract. 1 (1), 46–49.

Romanelli., G.G., Harper, R., Mock, D., et al., 1993. Evaluation of temporomandibular joint internal derangement. J. Orofac. Pain 7, 254.

Romanelli, G.G., Mock, D., Tenenbaum, H.C., 1992. Characteristics and response to treatment of posttraumatic temporomandibular disorder: A retrospective study. Clin. J. Pain 8, 6–17.

Straith, C.L., Lewis, J.R., 1948. Ankylosis of the temporomandibular joint. Plast. Reconstr. Surg. 3, 464–466.

Tenenbaum, H.C., Freeman, B.V., Psutka, D.J., Baker, G.I., 1999. Temporomandibular disorders: disk displacements. J. Orofacial Pain 13, 85–90.

Westesson, P.L., Bronstein, S.L., Liedberg, J., 1985. Internal derangement of the temporomandibular joint: morphologic description with correlation to joint function. Oral Surg. Oral Med. Oral Path. 59 (4), 323–331.

Wheeler, A.H., 2004. Myofascial pain disorders: theory to therapy. Drugs 64 (1), 45–62.

Yatani, H., Studts, J., Cordova, M., et al., 2002. Comparison of Sleep Quality and Clinical and Psychologic Characteristics in Patients with Temporomandibular Disorders. J. Orofacial Pain 16 (3), 221–228.

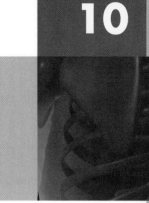

**10**

# PRINCIPLES OF JOINT AND PERIARTICULAR ASPIRATIONS AND INJECTIONS

Gillian A. Hawker • Elizabeth Grigoriadis • Adel G. Fam

## Indications for Aspiration and Injection of Joints and Periarticular Lesions

Aspiration and injection of joints and periarticular synovium-lined cavities (bursae and tendon sheaths) and injection of soft-tissue lesions (entheses, tendinitis, compression neuropathies, epidural sac) are indicated in the diagnosis and treatment of various musculoskeletal disorders. These are summarized in Table 10-1.

## Contraindications for Aspiration and Injection of Joints and Periarticular Lesions

The relative contraindications to intraarticular (IA) and periarticular injections of corticosteroids are summarized in Table 10–2. If infection is suspected in the joint, bursa, or tenosynovium, it should be aspirated and the synovial fluid examined for cell count, differential, and culture. In the setting of an inflamed joint, if the clinical diagnosis is unclear, or the aspirated fluid suggests possible infection, the aspirated fluid should be sent for cell count, differential, culture, and polarizing microscopy for crystals (Table 10-3). Intrasynovial corticosteroid injections may exacerbate an infection and are not recommended if there is suspicion of infection. Joint injection is also best avoided if there is bacteremia or infection of the overlying skin or subcutaneous tissue or in the presence of overlying skin lesions, such as extensive psoriatic plaques.

Bleeding disorders and severe thrombocytopenia are relative contraindications to joint aspiration. However, if diagnostic aspiration is deemed necessary, needle aspiration may be carried out after an appropriate cover for the bleeding disorder, such as factor VIII administration in a patient with hemophilia. Anticoagulant therapy with warfarin in the therapeutic range is not considered a contraindication to joint aspiration or injection.

Aspiration is recommended if prosthetic joint infection is suspected. However, a steroid injection into a prosthetic joint carries a particularly high risk of infection and is best avoided. Another risk is systemic absorption of a proportion of injected corticosteroid, which can result in worsening of uncontrolled diabetes mellitus, hypertension, congestive heart failure, or psychosis; such injections should be used cautiously in these patients.

## Complications of Intrasynovial and Periarticular Corticosteroid Injections

The potential complications of IA and intralesional corticosteroid injections are summarized in Table 10-4. The risk of **infection** after intrasynovial corticosteroid injections is very low; among practicing rheumatologists, one study documented the rate at less than 1 per 75,000 procedures, while

---

**TABLE 10-1**

### INDICATIONS FOR ASPIRATION AND INJECTION OF JOINTS AND PERIARTICULAR LESIONS

**Diagnosis**
Diagnostic synovial fluid analysis
   Septic arthritis, hemarthrosis, crystal arthritis, differentiation of inflammatory from noninflammatory arthritis
Diagnostic studies
   Arthrography
   Synovial biopsy
   Small-bore needle arthroscopy (needlescope)

**Therapy**
Repeated needle (closed) drainage of septic arthritis
Drainage of large hemorrhagic or tense effusions
Injection of therapeutic agents

*IA Corticosteroids*
Local control of inflammatory synovitis; periarticular lesions; efficacy in OA is less clear

*IA Hyaluronate Preparations*
Relief of pain in joints affected by OA

*IA Radioisotopes*
Control of chronic synovitis in inflammatory arthritis (radioactive synovectomy) using colloidal [198]gold (large joints), [90]yttrium (large joints), [186]rhenium (medium-sized joints), [169]erbium (small joints), and 32P chromic phosphate

(From Silva M, Luck JV Jr, Siegel ME. 32P chromic phosphate radiosynovectomy for chronic haemophilic synovitis. *Haemophilia* 2001;7 Suppl 2:40–49.)
IA, intraarticular; OA, osteoarthritis

127

a study of primary care practitioners in Britain prospectively documented no infections following 1147 steroid injections. Infection rates can be minimized by observing stringent aseptic "no-touch" techniques and by using sterile disposable needles and syringes and single-dose vials of corticosteroid and lidocaine. Local aspirations and injections can occasionally result in minor **hemorrhage** in the joint (hemarthrosis) or periarticular tissues (ecchymosis).

**Postinjection flare** is an acute, self-limiting, corticosteroid crystal–induced synovitis that may occur after IA or periarticular injections of insoluble, crystalline, intermediate- or long-acting corticosteroid preparations. It occurs in about 1% to 10% of patients, usually within 12 to 24 hours after injection. The reaction often resolves spontaneously in 48 to 72 hours, and the elbow, wrist, and finger joints are the most commonly affected sites. It is important to caution the patient that the joint may become more painful for up to 48 hours after the injection and that this flare is transient and does not affect the therapeutic outcome.

Repeated IA injection of large doses of corticosteroid into weight-bearing joints (e.g., knee, hip) may very rarely result in **joint deterioration,** disorganization, and instability that resembles a neuropathic arthropathy. This can be prevented by using small steroid doses and limiting the number of injections into the same joint to fewer than three to four injections per year.

---

### TABLE 10-2

### RELATIVE CONTRAINDICATIONS TO INTRAARTICULAR AND PERIARTICULAR CORTICOSTEROID INJECTIONS

Suspected joint infection
Overlying cellulitis or other skin infection
Systemic bacteremia
Thrombocytopenia, bleeding disorders
Prosthetic joints
Osteonecrosis, IA fracture or severely destroyed or unstable joint
Tendon tears and steroid injections near the Achilles tendon
Multiple or high-dose IA steroid injections in patients with uncontrolled diabetes mellitus, hypertension, congestive heart failure, or psychosis
Skin surface area covered by psoriatic plaques
Hypersensitivity to local anesthetic (steroid alone may be used)
Reluctant patient

IA, intraarticular

---

## SYSTEMIC EFFECTS

A certain degree of systemic absorption of steroid occurs after local injections. After IA injection, methylprednisolone acetate remains in the plasma for a mean of 16 days. This systemic absorption can result in a transient **steroid pulse**, with facial flushing, diaphoresis, and sometimes worsening of diabetic control and aggravation of hypertension, heart failure, or psychosis. It can also lead to both Cushing syndrome and suppression of the hypothalamic-pituitary-adrenal (HPA) axis, particularly in those receiving frequent large doses into multiple joints. This complication can be minimized by giving small, infrequent IA doses (fewer than three or four injections per year) and resting the joint for 24 to 48 hours after injection. Activity and exercise have been shown to increase the escape of steroids from the joint.

## LOCAL EFFECTS

Leakage of the steroid along the needle tract can lead to atrophy of both skin and subcutaneous fat, depigmentation, telangiectasia, and periarticular calcific deposits of hydroxyapatite crystals. This complication can be prevented by using a small-gauge needle and by applying local pressure for about 30 seconds after withdrawal of the needle.

**Misplaced needle injections** can lead to tendon rupture—particularly rotator cuff, long biceps, and Achilles tendons—nerve damage, injury of articular cartilage or IA disks, or formation of a sterile subcutaneous abscess or foreign-body granuloma.

# Technique of Joint Aspiration and Injection

## EQUIPMENT

Aspiration or injection of joints and soft tissues is an outpatient procedure that does not require specialized equipment. The equipment used includes povidone iodine or chlorhexidine, alcohol swabs, gauze pads, 1% or 2% lidocaine, ethyl chloride spray, disposable needles and syringes of various sizes, gloves, a corticosteroid preparation (Table 10-5), prepared small-patch dressing (e.g., Band-Aid), specimen bottles, and forceps.

---

### TABLE 10-3

### SYNOVIAL FLUID CHARACTERISTICS IN COMMON KNEE JOINT CONDITIONS

|  | **Normal** | **Osteoarthritis** | **Inflammatory Arthritis** | **Septic Arthritis** |
|---|---|---|---|---|
| Gross appearance | Clear | Clear | Cloudy or opaque | Opaque |
| Viscosity | High | High | Low | Low |
| Total synovial fluid WBC/mm$^3$ | < 200 | 200–1000 | 1,000–75,000 | > 50,000 |
| % Polymorphonuclear cells | < 25 | < 50 | > 50 | > 90 |
| Polarizing microscopy | Negative | Negative | Positive for crystals in gout or pseudogout | Negative |

## PROCEDURE

Using gloves, the clinician first identifies and marks the needle site with pressure from the cap of the needle and thoroughly cleanses the site with antiseptic solution or alcohol swabs. For local anesthesia, the skin and subcutaneous tissue are infiltrated down to the capsule with 1% or 2% lidocaine without epinephrine, using a small-bore needle. However, experienced physicians may opt to use topical anesthetics or no anesthetic at all; a single, quick needle thrust may be less painful than the local anesthetic when aspirating a joint effusion. With a proper aspiration technique, the needle passes freely through the skin, capsule, and synovial membrane, and a "pop" is felt as it enters the joint. Aspiration of synovial fluid confirms that the needle tip is within the joint space. If the fluid appearance raises any concerns about possible infection, injection should be abandoned and the fluid sent for cell count, differential, and culture. If the needle becomes clogged by fibrin clots, "rice bodies," or synovial villi, slight rotation or repositioning of the needle or reinjection of a little of the fluid will often help to unclog the needle and allow additional fluid to be aspirated. The aspirating syringe barrel is then detached with the aid of forceps, leaving the needle in place, and the steroid is injected through another syringe. The ease of injection determines whether the needle is in the joint space. If more than gentle pressure on the plunger is required to inject the steroid solution, the needle tip is probably not free in the synovial cavity and should be readjusted. At the end of the procedure, the needle is swiftly withdrawn, light pressure is applied with sterile gauze on the needle site for about 30 seconds, and a sterile Band-Aid is applied for a few hours.

The accuracy of outpatient IA and intralesional injections has recently come under close scrutiny. It is estimated that about 50% of IA and intralesional injections are placed incorrectly. Ultrasonographic or computed tomographic (CT) guidance of IA and periarticular aspirations and injections is particularly useful for injecting deep, inaccessible joints and for aspirating small amounts of fluid ($< 5$ mm$^3$). The procedure also reduces the risk of injury to articular cartilage, tendons, peripheral nerves, or blood vessels.

## FOLLOW-UP CARE

Resting an injected joint for 24 to 48 hours after an injection—particularly large, weight-bearing articulations—has been shown to reduce the escape of steroid from the joint and to improve the antiinflammatory response.

## PREPARATIONS OF INTRAARTICULAR AND PERIARTICULAR CORTICOSTEROID INJECTIONS

Corticosteroid preparations are divided into three categories based on potency and approximate duration of action of the drug (Table 10-6; see Table 10-5 also). **Hydrocortisone,** which can be synthesized, is the natural corticosteroid

---

| TABLE 10-4 |
| --- |
| **COMPLICATIONS OF INTRAARTICULAR AND INTRALESIONAL CORTICOSTEROID INJECTIONS** |

Introduction of infection
IA or periarticular hemorrhage
Postinjection flare
Destructive arthritis ("steroid arthropathy") from multiple IA injections into weight-bearing, partially damaged joints

**Systemic Effects**

Transient facial flush, warmth, and diaphoresis
Worsening of diabetic control, hypertension, heart failure, or psychosis
Suppression of HPA axis
Iatrogenic Cushing syndrome

**Local Effects**

Leakage of steroid along needle tract
Atrophy of subcutaneous fat, depigmentation, telangiectasia, and periarticular calcifications
Misplaced injections
Tendon rupture, nerve damage, cartilage injury, subcutaneous fat granuloma, and sterile abscess formation

**Rare Reactions**

Pancreatitis, hypersensitivity reactions, uterine bleeding, central serous chorioretinopathy, posterior subcapsular cataract, osteonecrosis

HPA, hypothalamic–pituitary–adrenal; IA, intraarticular

---

| TABLE 10-5 |
| --- |
| **PREPARATIONS OF INTRAARTICULAR AND PERIARTICULAR CORTICOSTEROIDS** |

| Preparation | Onset of Action | Duration of Action | Postinjection Flare |
| --- | --- | --- | --- |
| Short-acting (e.g., dexamethasone sodium [soluble] phosphate) | 1–2 hours | 12 days | None |
| Intermediate-acting (e.g., hydrocortisone acetate [Hydrocortone]) | 1–2 days | 1–4 weeks | Possible (insoluble) |
| Long-acting (e.g., methylprednisolone acetate [Depo-Medrol], triamcinolone acetonide [Kenalog], triamcinolone hexacetonide [Aristospan]) | 1–3 days | 2–4 months | Possible (insoluble) |

**TABLE 10-6**

## DOSAGES OF INTRAARTICULAR AND INTRALESIONAL CORTICOSTEROID INJECTIONS

| Drug | Large Joints (Knee, Hip, Shoulder) | Medium-Sized Joints (Elbow, Wrist, Ankle) | Small Joints (Hands and Feet) |
|---|---|---|---|
| Hydrocortisone acetate | 50–100 mg | 25–40 mg | 10–15 mg |
| Methylprednisolone acetate | 40–80 mg | 20–30 mg | 5–10 mg |
| Triamcinolone hexacetonide | 20–40 mg | 10–20 mg | 2.5–5 mg |

preparation. **Prednisolone** is less soluble, and the addition of methyl and acetate groups further reduces its solubility and prolongs its duration of action. The introduction of a fluorine atom to form **triamcinolone** enhances potency, and the addition of acetonide prolongs the duration of action. Therefore, the ranking order of potency is hydrocortisone, prednisolone salts, and then triamcinolone. Although triamcinolone is a highly effective preparation with a longer duration of action, it causes greater subcutaneous fat atrophy when leaked or injected extraarticularly compared to other steroid preparations. For this reason, use of prednisolone is preferred for periarticular injections.

## SELECTED READINGS

Berger, R.G., Yount, N.J., 1990. Immediate "steroid flare" from intra-articular triamcinolone hexacetonide injection: Case report and review of the literature. Arthritis Rheum. 33, 1284–1286.

Bernstein, R.M., 2001. Injections and surgical therapy in chronic pain. Clin. J. Pain 17, S94–S104.

Bird, H.A., 2003. Intra-articular and intralesional therapy. In: Hochberg, M.C., Silman, A.J., Smolen, J.S., et al (Eds.), Rheumatology, third ed. Mosby, Edinburgh, pp. 393–397.

Canoso, J.J., 2003. Aspiration and injection of joints and periarticular tissues. In: Hochberg, M.C., Silman, A.J., Smolen, J.S., et al (Eds.), Rheumatology, third ed. Mosby, Edinburgh, pp. 233–244.

Dieppe, P.A., Klippel, J.H., 1995. Aspiration and injection of joints and periarticular tissues. In: Klippel, J.H., Dieppe, P.A. (Eds.), Practical Rheumatology, first ed. Mosby, London, pp. 111–113.

Fam, A.G., 1995. The ankle and foot. In: Klippel, J.H., Dieppe, P.A. (Eds.), Practical Rheumatology, first ed. Mosby, London, pp. 120.

Grassi, W., Farina, A., Fillippucci, E., Cervini, C., 2001. Sonographically guided procedures in rheumatology. Semin. Arthritis Rheum. 30, 347–353.

Gray, R.C., Gottlieb, N.L., 1983. Intra-articular corticosteroids: An updated assessment. Clin. Orthop. 177, 235–263.

Jones, A., Regan, M., Ledingham, J., et al., 1993. Importance of placement of intra-articular steroid injection. Br. Med. J. 307, 1329–1330.

Kumar, N., Newman, R.J., 1999. Complications of intra- and peri-articular steroid injections. Br. J. Gen. Prac. 49, 465–466.

Pfenninger, J.L., 1991. Injections of joints and soft tissues. Part I: General guidelines. Am. Fam. Physician 44, 1196–1202.

Seror, P., Pluvinage, P., d'Andre, F.L., et al., 1999. Frequency of sepsis after local corticosteroid injection (an inquiry on 1,160,000 injections in rheumatological private practice in France). Rheumatology (Oxford) 38, 1272–1274.

Speed, C.A., 2001. Corticosteroid injections in tendon lesions. Br. Med. J. 323, 382–386.

# INDEX

Page numbers followed by f, t, or b indicate figures, tables, or boxes, respectively.